The Light of Yoga Society Beginner's Manual

Alice Christensen
and
David Rankin

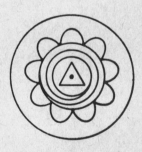

Simon and Schuster   New York

ISBN 0-671-21831-X
Manufactured in the United States of America

7   8   9   10   11   12   13   14

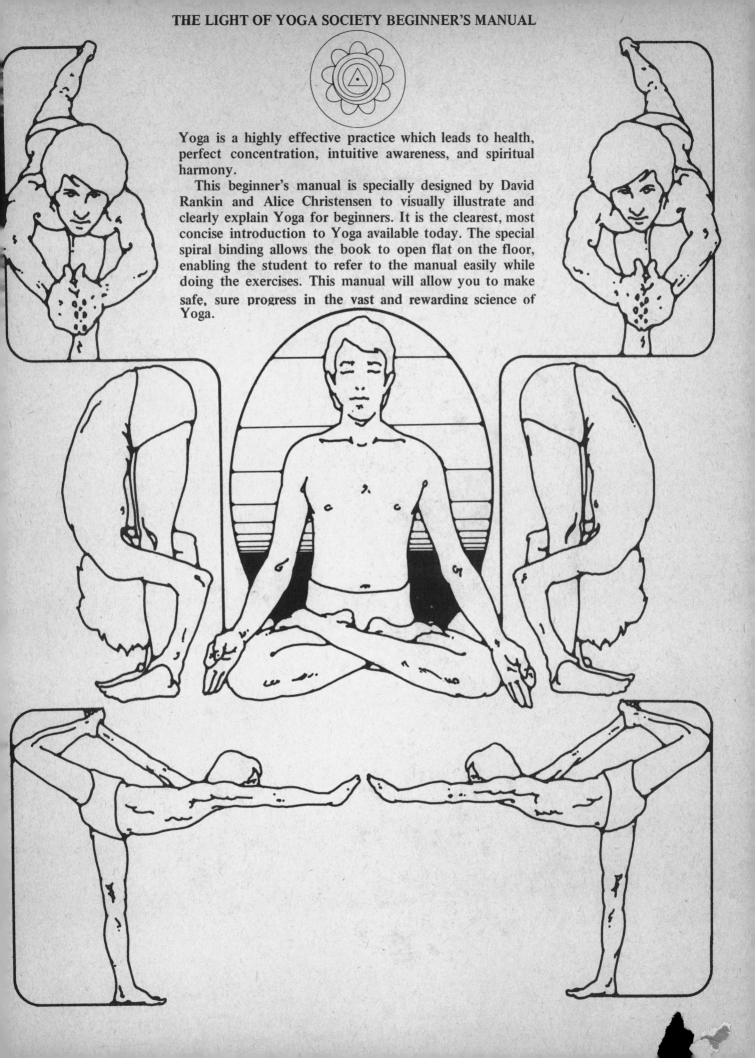

Yoga is a highly effective practice which leads to health, perfect concentration, intuitive awareness, and spiritual harmony.

This beginner's manual is specially designed by David Rankin and Alice Christensen to visually illustrate and clearly explain Yoga for beginners. It is the clearest, most concise introduction to Yoga available today. The special spiral binding allows the book to open flat on the floor, enabling the student to refer to the manual easily while doing the exercises. This manual will allow you to make safe, sure progress in the vast and rewarding science of Yoga.

This book is dedicated to the memory of our beloved Guru, Swami Rama. He came to us in love to enrich our lives, and to help The Light of Yoga Society teach Yoga in the Western world.

He was a firm believer in a safe, cautious approach to all the schools of Yoga, constantly stressing the perfect physical and mental balance one attains in Yoga when it is practiced slowly and correctly. It was this balance in his life which gave him the perfect illumination of a true master. Through his brilliance he was able to transcend the differences in Eastern and Western thought and to solidify the vast and complicated Vedantic wisdom into a practical, positive and effective means which enables man to find himself in this complex world.

This book was written under Swami Rama's direct supervision. The technique can be practiced by adults of every age to strengthen the nervous system and develop physical and mental health.

The bright light of perfection that shone through our Guru's teachings set a high standard for us here in the West. We will try to carry that light of great teaching with all the dignity, discipline, and respect that his memory deserves.

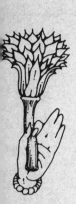

Alice Christensen began her Yoga practices in 1953, with an extraordinary vision of bright light which projected her into Yogic thought. She began a long correspondence with

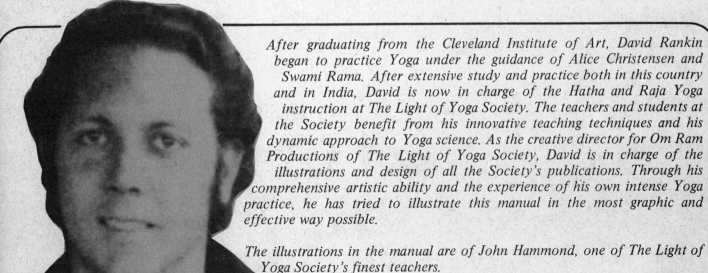

Swami Sivananda, Vedantic sage of Rishikesh, India, and with constant and sympathetic help proceeded strongly through her beginning disciplines of Yoga. Her Guru, Swami Rama, Raja Yoga master of Haridwar, India, came to take her to the Himalayas for advanced practices in 1964. Through her unequivocal devotion and the loving guidance of her teacher she has been able to explore the vast and brilliant world of Yoga. She returned to this country in 1965 and began to teach and lecture throughout the United States. Author of the book Light of Yoga, she frequently appears on radio and television presenting the enriching discipline of Yoga which changed her life. She was the first woman to lecture on Yoga at the University of New Delhi, and she accompanied her Guru, Swami Rama, as a delegate to the International Congress of Yoga in New Delhi, in 1970. She, David Rankin and a small group of dedicated students formed The Light of Yoga Society in that same year. She has said, "I did not consciously seek Yoga; rather it came to me and completely absorbed my whole life and thinking. Yoga has helped me attain that peace of mind, strength, inspiration, and energy which all of us need for living a full and complete life."

After graduating from the Cleveland Institute of Art, David Rankin began to practice Yoga under the guidance of Alice Christensen and Swami Rama. After extensive study and practice both in this country and in India, David is now in charge of the Hatha and Raja Yoga instruction at The Light of Yoga Society. The teachers and students at the Society benefit from his innovative teaching techniques and his dynamic approach to Yoga science. As the creative director for Om Ram Productions of The Light of Yoga Society, David is in charge of the illustrations and design of all the Society's publications. Through his comprehensive artistic ability and the experience of his own intense Yoga practice, he has tried to illustrate this manual in the most graphic and effective way possible.

The illustrations in the manual are of John Hammond, one of The Light of Yoga Society's finest teachers.

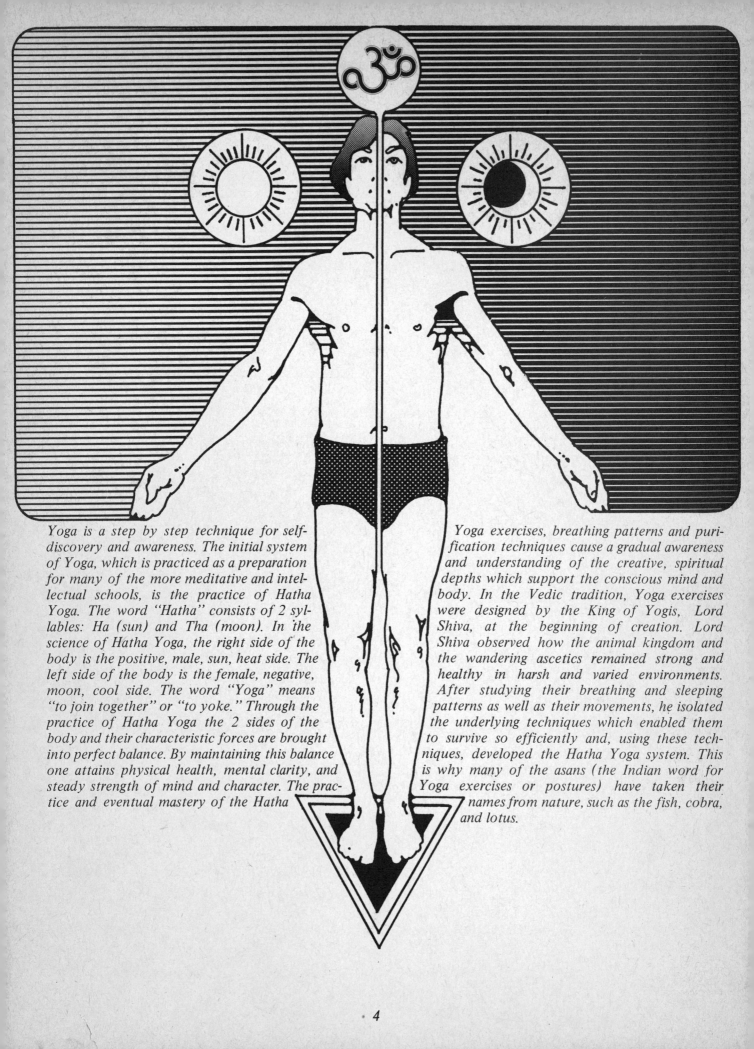

Yoga is a step by step technique for self-discovery and awareness. The initial system of Yoga, which is practiced as a preparation for many of the more meditative and intellectual schools, is the practice of Hatha Yoga. The word "Hatha" consists of 2 syllables: Ha (sun) and Tha (moon). In the science of Hatha Yoga, the right side of the body is the positive, male, sun, heat side. The left side of the body is the female, negative, moon, cool side. The word "Yoga" means "to join together" or "to yoke." Through the practice of Hatha Yoga the 2 sides of the body and their characteristic forces are brought into perfect balance. By maintaining this balance one attains physical health, mental clarity, and steady strength of mind and character. The practice and eventual mastery of the Hatha

Yoga exercises, breathing patterns and purification techniques cause a gradual awareness and understanding of the creative, spiritual depths which support the conscious mind and body. In the Vedic tradition, Yoga exercises were designed by the King of Yogis, Lord Shiva, at the beginning of creation. Lord Shiva observed how the animal kingdom and the wandering ascetics remained strong and healthy in harsh and varied environments. After studying their breathing and sleeping patterns as well as their movements, he isolated the underlying techniques which enabled them to survive so efficiently and, using these techniques, developed the Hatha Yoga system. This is why many of the asans (the Indian word for Yoga exercises or postures) have taken their names from nature, such as the fish, cobra, and lotus.

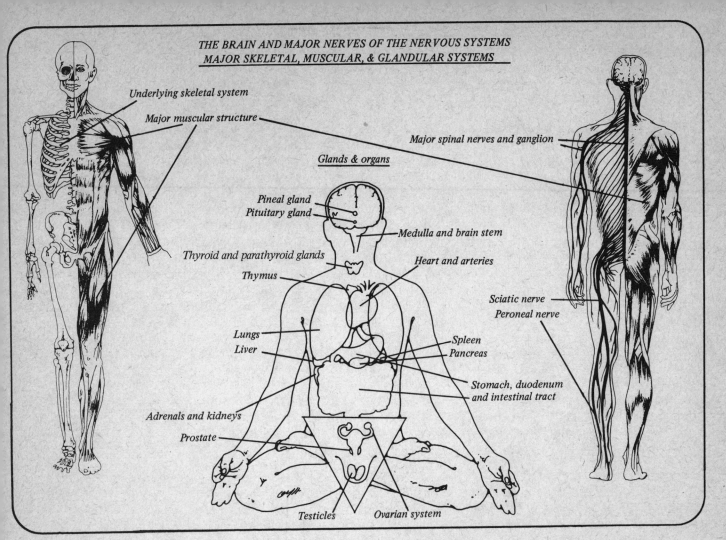

Underlying skeletal system
Major muscular structure
Major spinal nerves and ganglion
Glands & organs
Pineal gland
Pituitary gland
Medulla and brain stem
Thyroid and parathyroid glands
Heart and arteries
Thymus
Sciatic nerve
Peroneal nerve
Lungs
Spleen
Liver
Pancreas
Stomach, duodenum and intestinal tract
Adrenals and kidneys
Prostate
Testicles
Ovarian system

Yoga asans are designed to purify and give maximum flexibility and strength to the skeletal, muscular and nervous systems. The central nervous system is composed of the spinal cord and brain. The peripheral nervous system is made up of the motor and sensory nerves outside the central nervous system. The autonomic system is made up of the sympathetic and parasympathetic nervous systems and controls the unconscious and involuntary functions of the body and mind. Yoga exercise lays great stress on the effects of having a very supple, strong back and spinal column. The entire nervous system, central, peripheral and autonomic, is based in the spinal column. The thousands of nerves which control all organs and areas of the body can be traced back to the gigantic network of nerves in the spine and brain. We begin at the top of the spine and work throughout the body by stretching, twisting, balancing and breathing in a specifically designed manner. Through this process the vital organs are massaged and blood circulation is increased. This gentle, systematic pressure on the glands and vital organs causes hormones to be secreted which change the chemistry of the blood. This in turn causes a balanced, chemical change in the brain which alleviates tension and stress. This chemical change safely awakens normally inaccessible regions of the mind and brings about intuitive brilliance and creativity.

The primary concern of this manual is to allow the beginner to lay a firm, safe basis for further development of not only the physical exercises but, even more important, the mental and spiritual realms of Yoga practice. Most people have never considered that the exploration and control of the mind can be brought about by disciplined, physical exercise. The Hatha Yoga system has been designed to develop the intuitive, creative nature through the attainment of a dynamic balance of forces in the mind and body. This new awareness of the deep, inner resources of thought forms a substantial building block for the development of the entire personality.

According to Yogic science man's being is a microcosm which reflects the universe; the forces which compose the physical world are the same forces which operate the inner world. The understanding and mastery of the subtle and dynamic forces within the mind and body bring about a comprehension of the forces which create and control the universe. This understanding enables man to live in harmony with the macrocosm and arrive at a deeper awareness of his own divine self.

We have designed this manual to present the complex discipline of Yoga in a simple and understandable way. If you try to keep a few basic concepts in mind as you begin you will more easily receive the vast and enriching benefits of Yoga.

- *The first of these ideas to keep in mind is nonviolence (ahimsa). The general American conception of exercise as a strenuous competitive activity makes it difficult to correctly grasp the concept of passivity and gentleness employed in all of Yoga science. We have found in our years of teaching experience that most of those who are curious about Yoga should begin very gently and systematically. The intricate exercises and postures in Hatha Yoga need to be approached carefully with the proper state of mind. In Yoga you are not "whipping" the body into shape. Instead, you are trying to build a strong, healthy body and nervous system gradually and gracefully. Always move slowly as you get into a position and never strain or pull violently. Feel yourself flow from one position to the next and don't be discouraged if you don't seem to be progressing as rapidly as you think you should. It takes time for the body to become limber and it is far better to go as far as you can comfortably than to try to force yourself into a completed position prematurely. Remember that Yoga exercise is done to rest rather than exhaust the body; therefore, you should try to practice your exercises smoothly and nonviolently. There should never be any idea of competition or negativity in your mind as you practice the asans.*

- *The second concept is to use common sense as you approach Yoga. Never exceed your limitations. If you have had an operation recently or have a physical disability, please check with your doctor before trying to practice any of the exercises in this manual. If you are elderly or have high blood pressure you need to use even more caution as you exercise. Do not begin by doing exercises that are too demanding or difficult; start slowly and work up to the difficult asans as you progress. Realize that some parts of the body will be stiffer than others and therefore need special care and attention. You will also notice that you will be stiffer in the morning than in the evening.*

  Always remember that Yoga is balanced. Most people find one side of the body more limber than the other. Use caution when exercising the stiff side and always try to maintain a pose for the same time in both directions. This helps to bring about an equalization of the complementary forces in each side of the body and mind. Never let your desire to succeed override your common sense. If there is any discomfort either while holding a position or afterward you are working too hard. It says in the Bhagavad Gita (18 Chapters of Yoga by Lord Krishna) that "Yoga is not for the glutton or for one who fasts too much. It is not for the sleepheavy or the sleepless. Yoga destroys despair; it is only for the moderate in eating and resting, in sleeping and working." Therefore, use your common sense as you approach Yoga. If you proceed moderately with an awareness of your own capabilities and limitations you will be far more successful and much happier than if you attempt too much too soon.

- *The third idea to try to remember is that these Yoga asans have an effect on the mind. If you ignore this dimension of your practices you will certainly become healthy but you will have missed the real treasure of Yoga discipline. Try to control your thoughts as you exercise. Concentrate on what you are doing. You are trying to realize how beautiful and happy you really are and your Yoga practice will bring about this realization. Concentrate on the rhythm of your breathing. This will help still the mind and prevent distracting thoughts from disturbing your concentration. Those who practice Yoga are trying to produce harmony and balance in themselves and the world and it is this dimension of mental growth within Yoga that brings this about.*

- *One of the most important points is to be regular in your practices. All too often students try to work too hard for the first six months and find themselves incapable of supporting the massive amount of discipline they have taken on. Yoga is not a burden; it is something you should enjoy, but like anything else it takes an initial commitment and dedication before it becomes really satisfying. The best way to proceed is to set aside about fifteen or twenty minutes a day for your Yoga practices and then try to stick to it. More often than not in the beginning there will be some days when you just don't have twenty minutes to do a complete routine of exercise, but even on these days, find the time to do a few positions. (See page 56 for a quick routine.) You are trying to develop concentration and will-power—keeping regular in your disciplines is perhaps the most important facet of that process. Don't let yourself fabricate excuses to keep you from doing your disciplines and don't allow yourself to become discouraged. Progress in Yoga comes through systematic daily discipline. If you work every day for four or five weeks you will be amazed at how far you will progress. Remember: if you are rushed or busy and can't find time to do your complete Yoga routine do some portion of your discipline. It is this commitment to daily practice that will stabilize both your mind and your emotions.*

● *The final point we wish to emphasize is to read this manual thoroughly. Read the text of an asan before you attempt to do it and reread the "Cautions and Hints" and "Benefits of the Asans" (in the back of the manual) and the basic text frequently. We recommend that you follow the beginners program located on page 56. This program is designed around our class structure which lasts approximately six weeks. If you are not in a class it may take you eight to ten weeks to complete this program. If you are working on your own, proceed carefully at your own pace, but make sure that as you progress you continue to work on more challenging asans. If you do not have time to do a full program, follow the abbreviated routine on page 56 which provides the essential stretches to the spine.*

You may want to take a break during your work day to relax with Yoga. All of the warm-ups and standing poses are excellent for removing fatigue and tension and will help clear the mind. All of these can be done in an office or a coffee break or lunch hour. Taking a Yoga break instead of a coffee break will increase your energy and work output, relieve stress, and make you peaceful and balanced-minded.

This book was designed to afford maximum benefit and efficiency to the beginner in Yoga. The special spiral binding will allow you to lay the manual flat on the floor in front of you so that you can follow it very easily. Rather than demonstrate the exercises with only an illustration of the completed posture and a lengthy description, we have tried to show in simple design and illustration a practical and concise way of approaching the various positions. If you follow carefully the arrows and illustrations with the accompanying text you will be successful in gaining excellent benefits from your practices. If you are able to work with a properly disciplined teacher at the same time, so much the better. When doing your Yoga, please remember to keep these five basic ideas in mind as you begin.

● *Approach your practices gently and nonviolently.*

● *Use common sense.*

● *Do your practices every day.*

● *Follow the manual and reread it frequently.*

● *Watch the effect that asans have on your mind and body.*

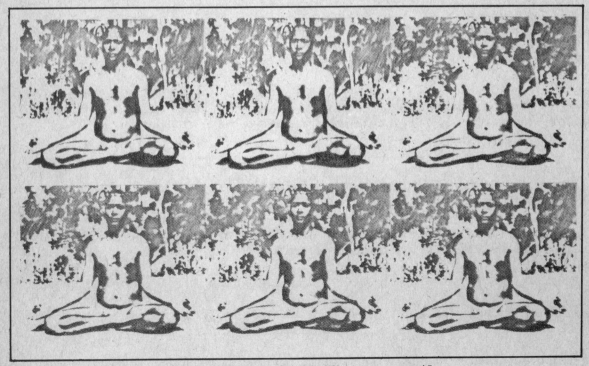

Swami Rama seated in Siddhasan at age 45.

CAUTIONS AND HINTS

Read these suggestions before you start to exercise and go back to them periodically to gain the most from your Yoga practice.

- *Read the text of the different poses before attempting them. Then try the exercise itself and go back and read the text again.*

- *Use a blanket or mat to do your Yoga practices. Keep this blanket and your exercise clothes separate for your Yoga practice only. This will help to stabilize your mental and emotional nature.*

- *Do not do these exercises in a cold, drafty area; warmth is very important.*

- *If you do these exercises after work, a quick shower before you begin will help wash off the upsetting vibrations of the day and make for a more rewarding experience and effectiveness in your practices.*

- *Always use caution, common sense and gentleness in these exercises.*

- *Always move slowly, passively and smoothly in these exercises.*

- *At no time should you bounce, jerk, twist or bend quickly or uncontrollably as you practice.*

- *Never do these asans while under the influence of hallucinogens, narcotics, barbiturates or alcohol.*

- *Do not do asans for at least 2½ hours after eating.*

- *Do not drink coffee, tea or alcohol for at least 1½ hours before exercising as this may upset the heart and blood pressure. Tea with milk, however, can be taken 45 minutes beforehand.*

- *Three repetitions is all that is recommended for most of these asans except where otherwise specified. These exercises are not like calisthenics, where the more repetition, the more effect is produced. Yoga creates the maximum benefit through the minimum expenditure of energy.*

- *At no time should you hold your breath in or out for more than 5 to 10 seconds in any of the asans shown in this manual.*

- *Do not try to do the advanced headstand (which is not shown in this manual) or the complicated breathing exercises of Yoga, pranayamas, unless you are working closely with a highly qualified instructor. There are many strict prerequisites which must be followed closely before attempting these practices.*

- *Always breathe through the nose in doing these exercises. For the best effect, the breath should flow through both nostrils evenly. In advanced practices this becomes quite important.*

- *As you breathe in, feel your body filling with energy, light, health and happiness.*

- *As you breathe out, feel all of the impurities, illnesses, negativity, hatred and violence leave your body and mind.*

- *After every 2 or 3 asans, you should rest and relax completely for 30 to 60 seconds in Savasan (corpse pose) (60A), Virasan (33A, B), or the Easy Bridge Rest (32A).*

- *In exercises where the eyes are to be focused on a specific point for a length of time, do not strain.*

- *When balancing on one leg or trying to hold a certain position for a length of time, fix the gaze on one spot. This will strengthen the eyes and concentration and will still the mind.*

- *Do not do these exercises during pregnancy or the menstrual period. (Some people say it is all right to do these exercises during these times; however, there are too many complications and injuries that could take place unless you are working under the very strict and close observation of a highly qualified instructor.)*

- *Do not try to impress your friends with your accomplishments as this may cause physical and mental barriers to further progress.*

- *Do not try to force your practices on other people. Become established in your practices and let the results speak for themselves.*

- *Try to develop a calm, quiet mental attitude while doing your asans. Be careful not to dwell on depressing or violent thoughts or troubles during your practices as the thoughts and problems will take on greater proportions.*

- *Be calm, positive, and confident at all times.*

- *Do not allow minor setbacks to discourage you.*

- *If you are elderly, proceed carefully and be very gentle with yourself.*

- *Be firm with yourself in doing your exercises daily. Do not allow your mind to create unnecessary or imaginary reasons for not sticking with your practices.*

- *The best time to do your exercises is whenever you can find quiet, undisturbed time. Some people find it best to do their practices in the early morning; in that way the mind and body are toned up for the day ahead. Others find the time during lunch hour appropriate for it helps them to refresh and recharge. Other people find that doing their practices at the end of the day after work helps them to unwind, relieve stress and to relax. Choose the time that fits best into your schedule.*

- *Minor aches and soreness develop in most any exercise when one is out of shape. Beginners should not be alarmed by this. If, however, you notice headaches, muscle strain, nerve strain, uncommon nervousness and irritability, bleeding, cramps, dislocations, fainting or dizziness, or similar upsets, then something you are doing is incorrect. Perhaps you are trying too hard, straining, or you may have some physical problem which should be evaluated more carefully.*

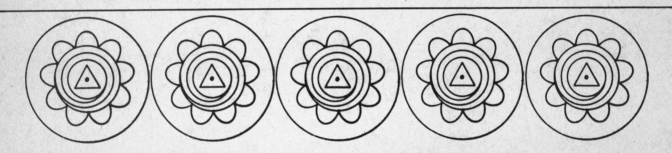

Many people are teaching Yoga in the United States today. You may be able to find classes in high schools, colleges, YMCAs, church groups, etc. Some of the instructors are qualified, many are not. Question your instructor about his own Yoga practice and conduct. Find out about his teachers and his relationship with them. A genuine teacher has allowed Yoga to influence his entire life style. His dedication and devotion to his own disciplines and teachers gives you some idea of the quality of the instruction you are receiving.

In The Light of Yoga Society, a teacher is required to observe the spiritual and ethical guidelines given to us by our Guru, Shri Swami Rama, and his disciple, Alice Christensen. A teacher for The Light of Yoga Society is disciplined in body and mind. This discipline includes daily meditation and puja (worship); extensive daily mantric Yoga practice (continuous repetition of God's name with a conscious effort to assimilate divine qualities); and daily practice of Yoga exercise (Hatha Yoga). In addition, a teacher must possess an accurate understanding of the principles, philosophy and mythologies of Yoga as well as a practical knowledge of nutrition. The teachers must also conduct themselves in accordance with Yogic precepts, which include the practice of nonviolence (yamas and niyamas) and strict vegetarianism. A teacher must also observe complete abstinence from smoking and, of course, from all hallucinogens and narcotics. Most importantly, however, the members of The Light of Yoga Society's teaching staff are dedicated and sincere about their Yoga practices and all of them are making an active, devoted attempt to establish themselves in a well-rounded spiritual discipline.

HEAD ROTATIONS: *To begin Yoga exercise we always recommend that one should warm-up the nerves, muscles and circulation of the body before attempting to do anything in the way of strenuous stretching or balancing. The exercises on the first several pages of this book are designed to increase circulation, limber up the spine, and warm-up the muscles, tendons and nerves. The first exercise is called the Head Roll. This is done in four basic movements. First (1A), the right ear is lowered to the right shoulder, as the arms are outstretched, palms up. Next (1B), the head is lowered backwards, then (1C), the left ear is lowered to the left shoulder, and lastly (1D), the face comes forward, with the chin to the chest.*

(1A)

(1B)

After you become familiar with these four basic positions, proceed to gently roll the head in a 360° circle (1E), smoothly going from one position to the next. Then, reverse the process, rotating the head in the opposite direction (3 rotations to the left, 3 rotations to the right).

Most people in the beginning will notice some grinding sounds in the neck. This is due to a lack of proper exercise and many times to a calcium deficiency in one's diet. In a few weeks you will notice improvement in the mobility and strength of the neck.

(1C)

CAUTION: *This exercise should not be done if one has neck injuries.*

(1D)

360°

(1E)

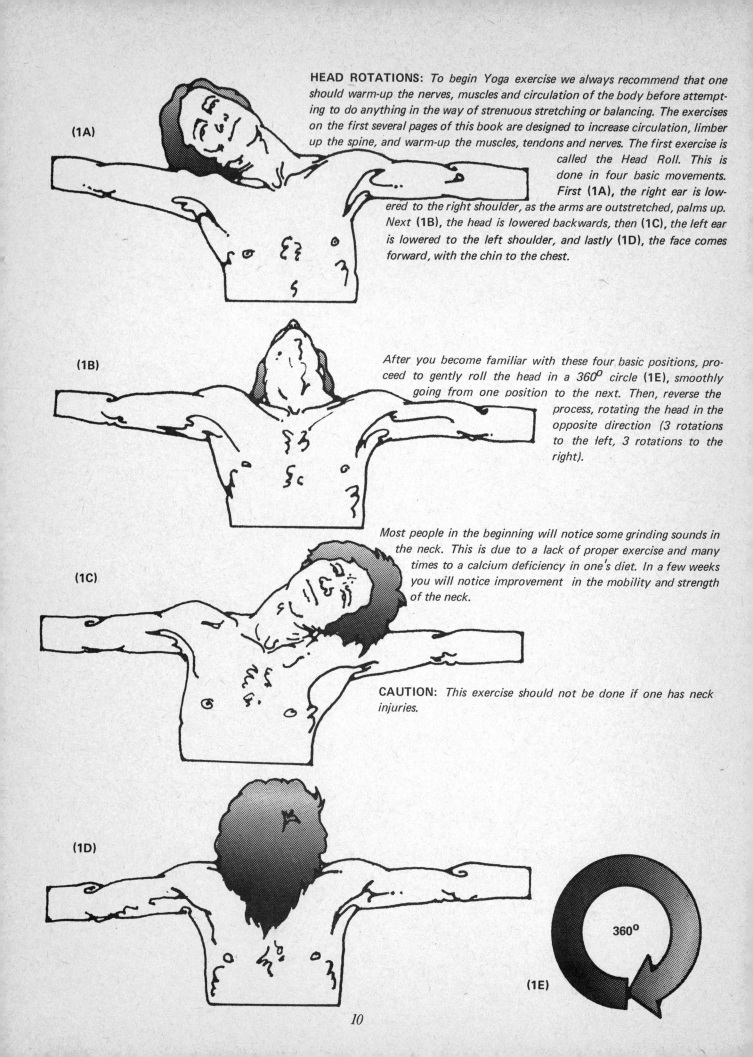

10

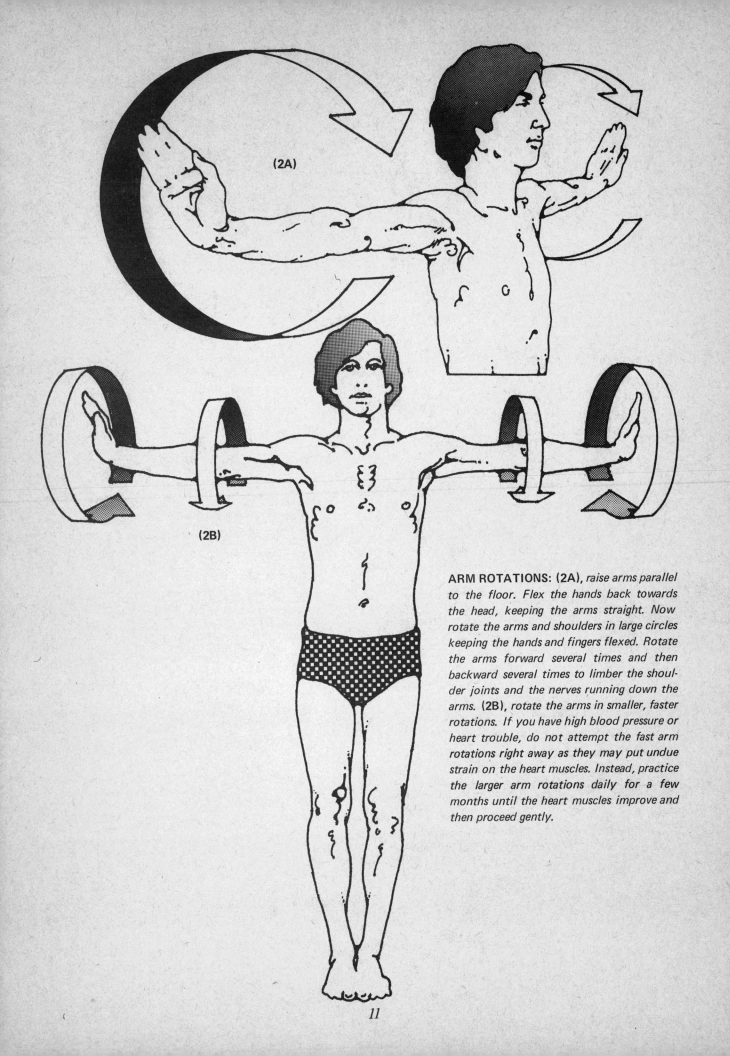

ARM ROTATIONS: (2A), *raise arms parallel to the floor. Flex the hands back towards the head, keeping the arms straight. Now rotate the arms and shoulders in large circles keeping the hands and fingers flexed. Rotate the arms forward several times and then backward several times to limber the shoulder joints and the nerves running down the arms. (2B), rotate the arms in smaller, faster rotations. If you have high blood pressure or heart trouble, do not attempt the fast arm rotations right away as they may put undue strain on the heart muscles. Instead, practice the larger arm rotations daily for a few months until the heart muscles improve and then proceed gently.*

(2A)

(2B)

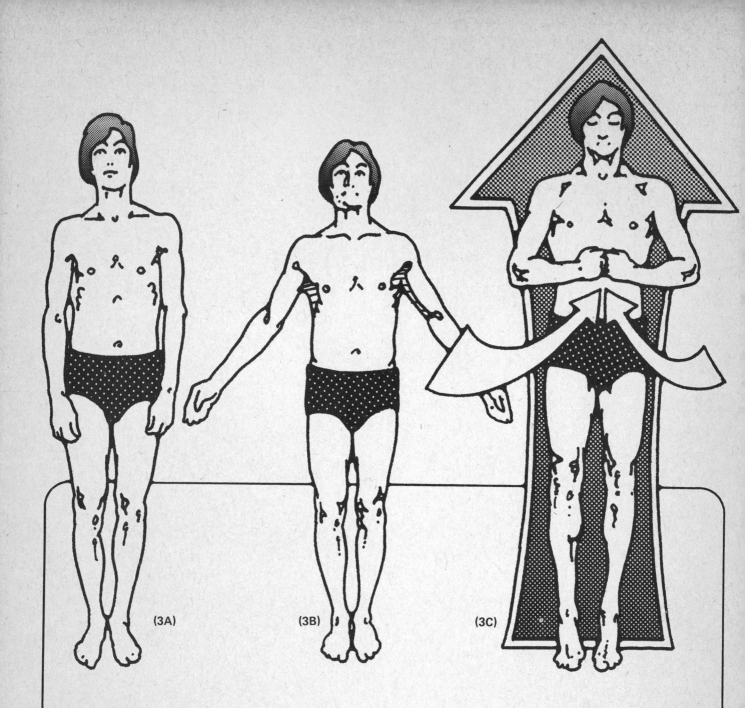

(3A)   (3B)   (3C)

RAMA'S EASY POSE (1): *This is a simple exercise but very effective in warming up the nervous system in the entire body.* **(3A),** *stand erect with your arms to the sides and exhale through the nose.* **(3B),** *extend arms slightly to the sides, and begin to inhale slowly and deeply through the nose as you rise off the floor onto the toes.* **(3C),** *as you rise, make fists of your hands and pull the fists tight into the chest just below the ribcage. Hold this Position* **(3C),** *with your lungs filled with air while standing on the toes. Do not let the eyes wander. Rather, fix the gaze on one spot. This will help you keep your balance. Try to hold the breath 5 to 10 seconds, then slowly begin to exhale, lowering the heels to the floor, and allowing the arms to relax at the sides. Repeat this asan 3 times.*

This exercise helps chronic constipation and strengthens the ankles, feet, and legs. It also helps to strengthen the eyes and makes them clear and bright.

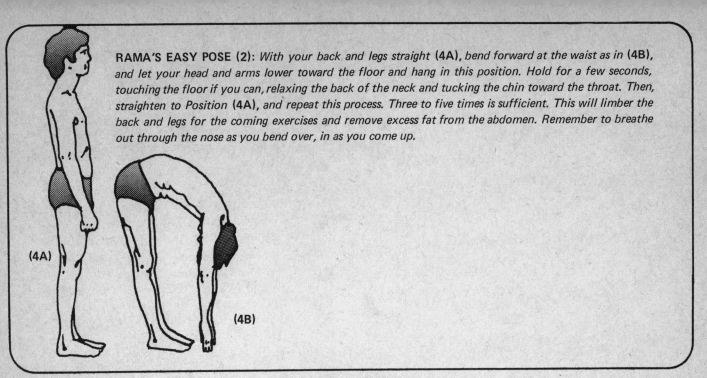

RAMA'S EASY POSE (2): *With your back and legs straight* **(4A)**, *bend forward at the waist as in* **(4B)**, *and let your head and arms lower toward the floor and hang in this position. Hold for a few seconds, touching the floor if you can, relaxing the back of the neck and tucking the chin toward the throat. Then, straighten to Position* **(4A)**, *and repeat this process. Three to five times is sufficient. This will limber the back and legs for the coming exercises and remove excess fat from the abdomen. Remember to breathe out through the nose as you bend over, in as you come up.*

(4A)

(4B)

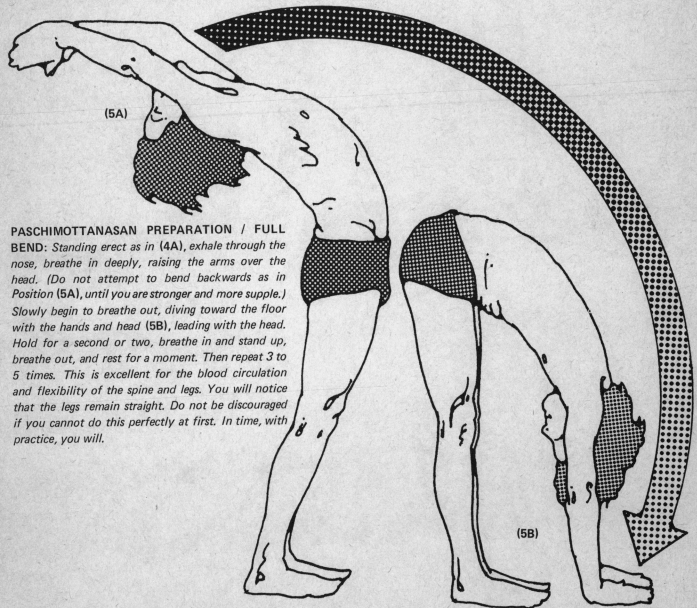

(5A)

PASCHIMOTTANASAN PREPARATION / FULL BEND: *Standing erect as in* **(4A)**, *exhale through the nose, breathe in deeply, raising the arms over the head. (Do not attempt to bend backwards as in Position* **(5A)**, *until you are stronger and more supple.) Slowly begin to breathe out, diving toward the floor with the hands and head* **(5B)**, *leading with the head. Hold for a second or two, breathe in and stand up, breathe out, and rest for a moment. Then repeat 3 to 5 times. This is excellent for the blood circulation and flexibility of the spine and legs. You will notice that the legs remain straight. Do not be discouraged if you cannot do this perfectly at first. In time, with practice, you will.*

(5B)

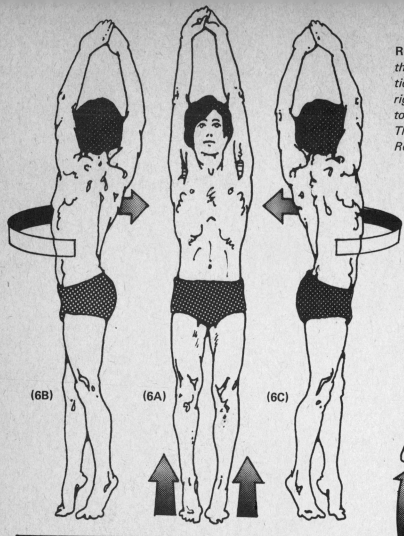

(6B) **(6A)** **(6C)**

RAMA'S EASY POSE TWIST: *Stand straight with arms at the side, exhale, breathe in, rise up on the toes as in Position* **(6A)**, *holding the breath. Now, gently twist to the right and look behind as far as possible* **(6B)**. *Then, return to* **(6A)**, *exhale slowly, lower heels to the floor and relax. Then, inhale, rise again* **(6A)**, *and twist to the left* **(6C)**. *Repeat this process once or twice in each direction.*

COMPLETE LEG LIFT: *Start with both hands on the hips and lift the left leg straight in front* **(8A)**. *Now, holding the foot in the air, swing the leg around to* **(8B)**. *Then continue to* **(8C)**, *holding momentarily at each position. Try not to bend forward. Lower the left leg to the floor and repeat with the right leg (1 to 2 repetitions with each leg). If your balance is unsteady, do not hesitate to lean on the back of a chair. This exercise will give good muscle tone to hips and a nice, flat stomach and diaphragm.*

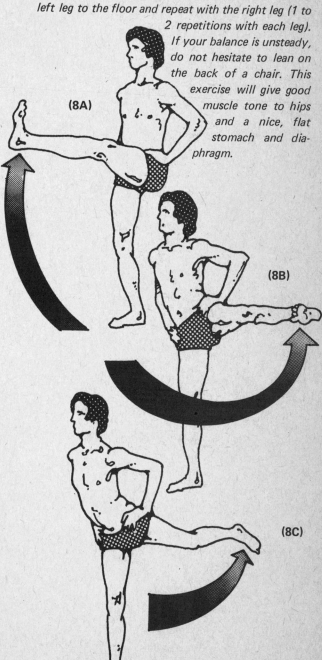

(8A)

(8B)

(8C)

ALTERNATE LEG LIFT: **(7A)**, *stand erect with the right hand on the right hip and raise the left arm out parallel to the floor. Then lift the left leg up with the foot flexed toward the head until the toes touch the fingers. Keep the leg straight. Lower the leg slowly. Repeat 3 to 5 times to each leg. Keep the knees as straight as possible, as this will lengthen the tendons in the leg.*

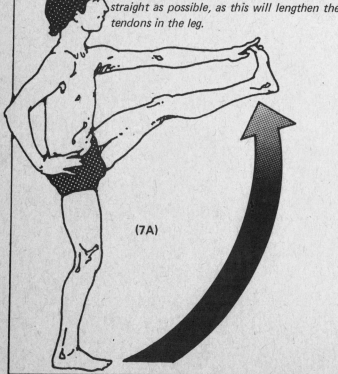

(7A)

14

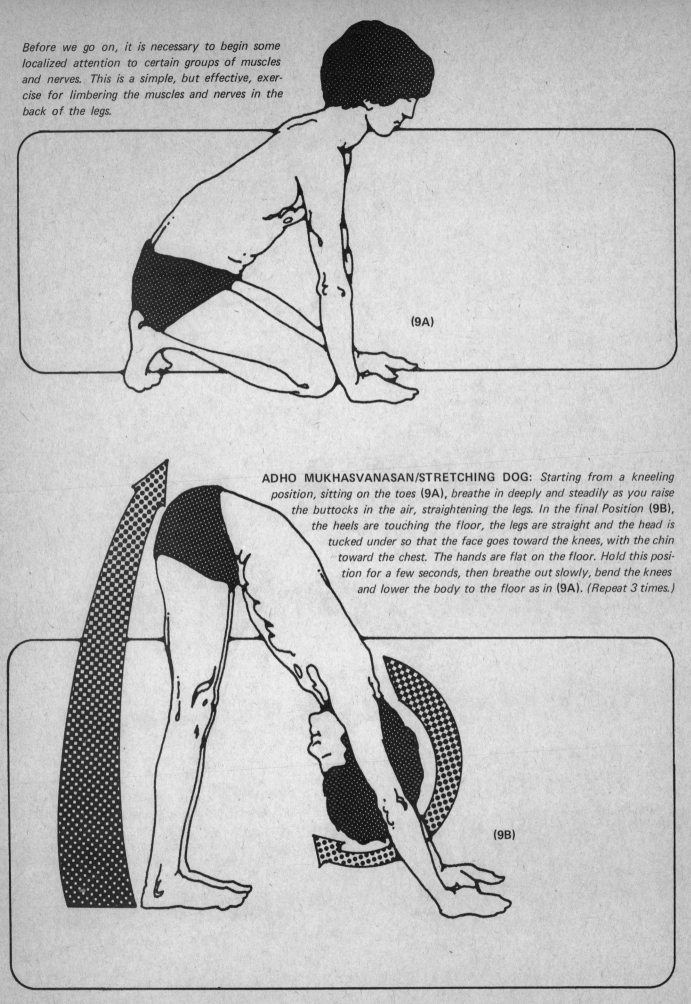

Before we go on, it is necessary to begin some localized attention to certain groups of muscles and nerves. This is a simple, but effective, exercise for limbering the muscles and nerves in the back of the legs.

(9A)

ADHO MUKHASVANASAN/STRETCHING DOG: *Starting from a kneeling position, sitting on the toes* **(9A)**, *breathe in deeply and steadily as you raise the buttocks in the air, straightening the legs. In the final Position* **(9B)**, *the heels are touching the floor, the legs are straight and the head is tucked under so that the face goes toward the knees, with the chin toward the chest. The hands are flat on the floor. Hold this position for a few seconds, then breathe out slowly, bend the knees and lower the body to the floor as in* **(9A)**. *(Repeat 3 times.)*

(9B)

The spine is now becoming more limber and you may begin to feel which muscles and nerves in the legs and spine are in need of more flexibility and strength. These next few exercises give great benefit to a nervous system and brain that are under severe pressure or stress.

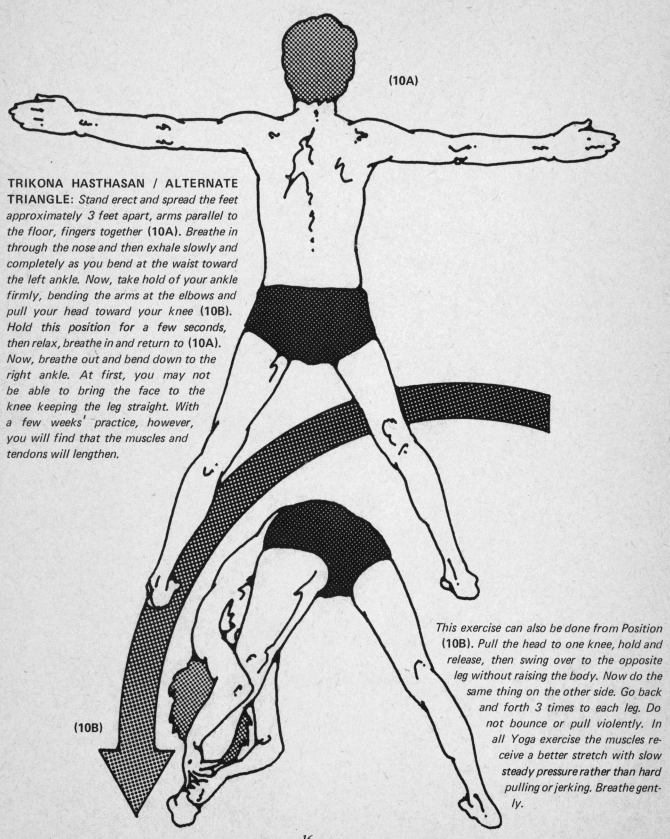

(10A)

TRIKONA HASTHASAN / ALTERNATE TRIANGLE: *Stand erect and spread the feet approximately 3 feet apart, arms parallel to the floor, fingers together (10A). Breathe in through the nose and then exhale slowly and completely as you bend at the waist toward the left ankle. Now, take hold of your ankle firmly, bending the arms at the elbows and pull your head toward your knee (10B). Hold this position for a few seconds, then relax, breathe in and return to (10A). Now, breathe out and bend down to the right ankle. At first, you may not be able to bring the face to the knee keeping the leg straight. With a few weeks' practice, however, you will find that the muscles and tendons will lengthen.*

(10B)

This exercise can also be done from Position (10B). Pull the head to one knee, hold and release, then swing over to the opposite leg without raising the body. Now do the same thing on the other side. Go back and forth 3 times to each leg. Do not bounce or pull violently. In all Yoga exercise the muscles receive a better stretch with slow steady pressure rather than hard pulling or jerking. Breathe gently.

16

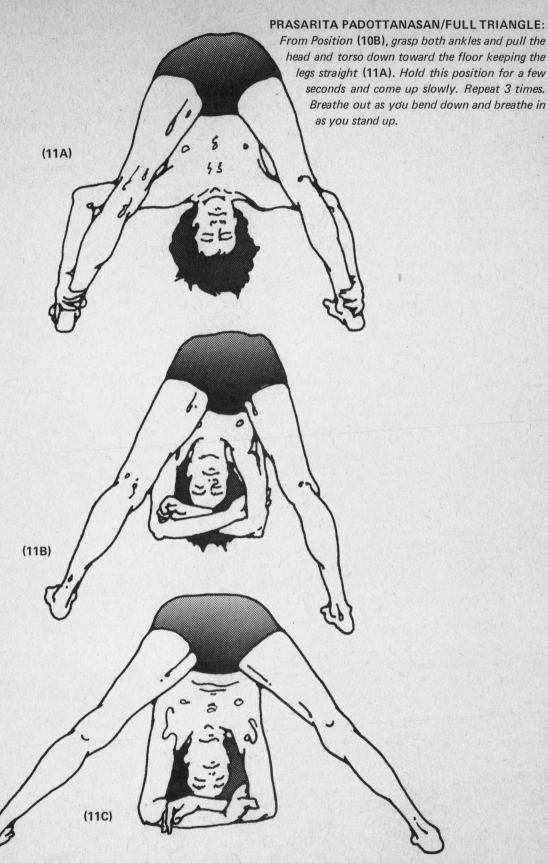

PRASARITA PADOTTANASAN/FULL TRIANGLE:
From Position **(10B)**, *grasp both ankles and pull the head and torso down toward the floor keeping the legs straight* **(11A)**. *Hold this position for a few seconds and come up slowly. Repeat 3 times. Breathe out as you bend down and breathe in as you stand up.*

(11A)

(11B)

(11C)

(11B, C) *are more difficult and may take some time to achieve.* **(11B)**, *interlock the arms and hold this position for several seconds. In* **(11C)**, *the feet are stretched further apart and the head and arms rest on the floor. The legs remain completely straight. This stretches the interior thigh muscles considerably. When you can do this asan perfectly, you have become limber enough to go on to more advanced asans. Breathe normally in* **(11B, C)**.

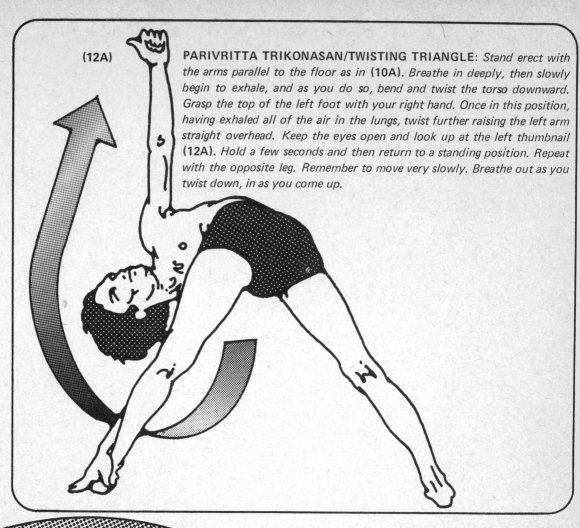

(12A)

PARIVRITTA TRIKONASAN/TWISTING TRIANGLE: *Stand erect with the arms parallel to the floor as in* **(10A)**. *Breathe in deeply, then slowly begin to exhale, and as you do so, bend and twist the torso downward. Grasp the top of the left foot with your right hand. Once in this position, having exhaled all of the air in the lungs, twist further raising the left arm straight overhead. Keep the eyes open and look up at the left thumbnail* **(12A)**. *Hold a few seconds and then return to a standing position. Repeat with the opposite leg. Remember to move very slowly. Breathe out as you twist down, in as you come up.*

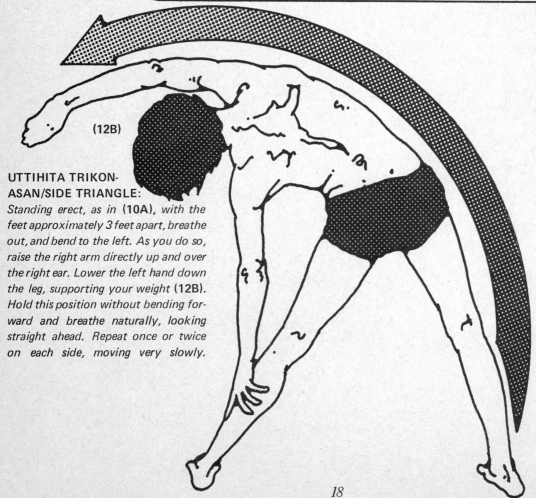

(12B)

UTTIHITA TRIKON-ASAN/SIDE TRIANGLE:

Standing erect, as in **(10A)**, *with the feet approximately 3 feet apart, breathe out, and bend to the left. As you do so, raise the right arm directly up and over the right ear. Lower the left hand down the leg, supporting your weight* **(12B)**. *Hold this position without bending forward and breathe naturally, looking straight ahead. Repeat once or twice on each side, moving very slowly.*

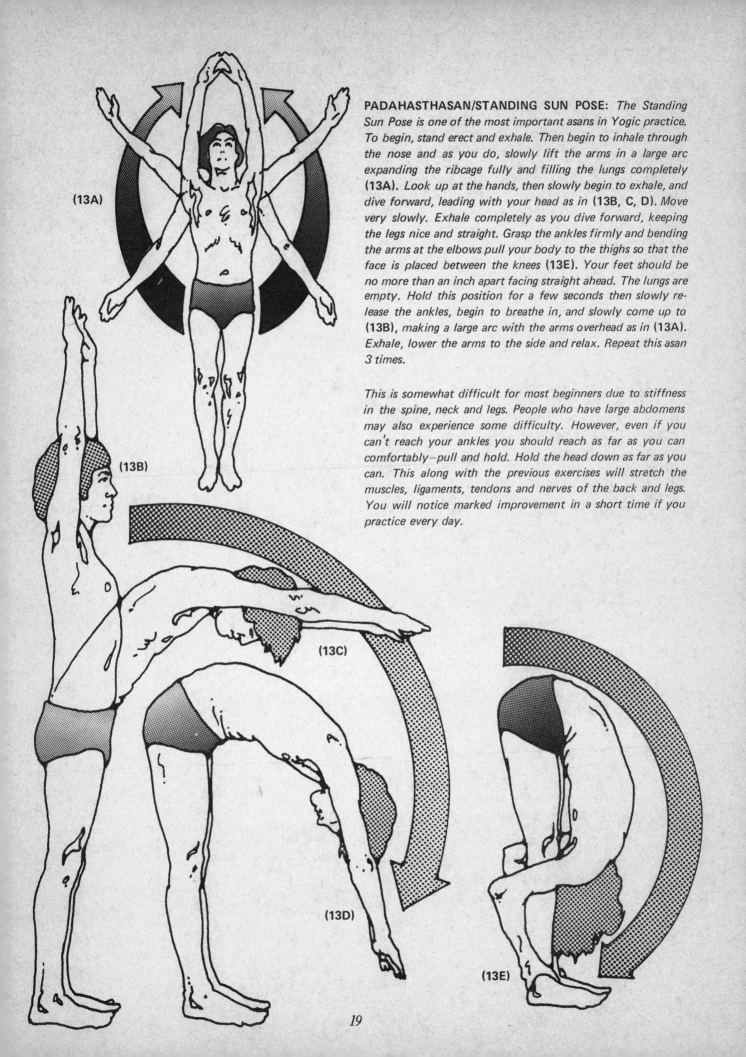

(13A)

(13B)

(13C)

(13D)

(13E)

PADAHASTHASAN/STANDING SUN POSE: *The Standing Sun Pose is one of the most important asans in Yogic practice. To begin, stand erect and exhale. Then begin to inhale through the nose and as you do, slowly lift the arms in a large arc expanding the ribcage fully and filling the lungs completely* **(13A)**. *Look up at the hands, then slowly begin to exhale, and dive forward, leading with your head as in* **(13B, C, D)**. *Move very slowly. Exhale completely as you dive forward, keeping the legs nice and straight. Grasp the ankles firmly and bending the arms at the elbows pull your body to the thighs so that the face is placed between the knees* **(13E)**. *Your feet should be no more than an inch apart facing straight ahead. The lungs are empty. Hold this position for a few seconds then slowly release the ankles, begin to breathe in, and slowly come up to* **(13B)**, *making a large arc with the arms overhead as in* **(13A)**. *Exhale, lower the arms to the side and relax. Repeat this asan 3 times.*

This is somewhat difficult for most beginners due to stiffness in the spine, neck and legs. People who have large abdomens may also experience some difficulty. However, even if you can't reach your ankles you should reach as far as you can comfortably—pull and hold. Hold the head down as far as you can. This along with the previous exercises will stretch the muscles, ligaments, tendons and nerves of the back and legs. You will notice marked improvement in a short time if you practice every day.

PARSVOTTANASAN/STANDING SUN POSE VARIATION: *We have added this variation of the Padahasthasan for those of you who are rather limber and can do a more challenging pose. As you can see from* **(14A)**, *the hands are clasped and interlocked behind the back, and the arms are straightened and flexed up and away from the body. This manner of flexing the arms behind the back is common to several other advanced Yoga asans. It is very beneficial in that it lubricates and limbers the shoulder joints, upper back muscles and lumbar vertebrae. Even more importantly, it expands and stretches the ribcage and lungs which allows fresh blood and energy into the nerves and tissues of the lungs, chest, heart, etc. This asan should not be attempted until proficiency has been gained in the standing Padahasthasan* **(13E).**

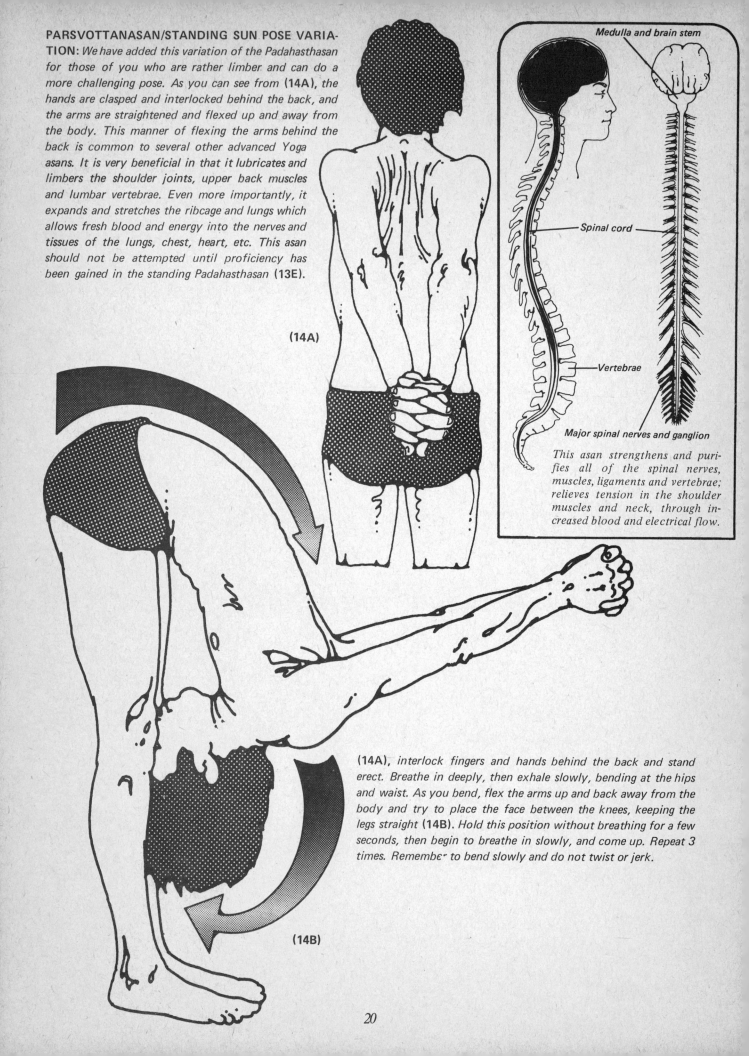

(14A)

Medulla and brain stem

Spinal cord

Vertebrae

Major spinal nerves and ganglion

This asan strengthens and purifies all of the spinal nerves, muscles, ligaments and vertebrae; relieves tension in the shoulder muscles and neck, through increased blood and electrical flow.

(14A), *interlock fingers and hands behind the back and stand erect. Breathe in deeply, then exhale slowly, bending at the hips and waist. As you bend, flex the arms up and back away from the body and try to place the face between the knees, keeping the legs straight* **(14B)**. *Hold this position without breathing for a few seconds, then begin to breathe in slowly, and come up. Repeat 3 times. Remember to bend slowly and do not twist or jerk.*

(14B)

VRIKSASAN/TREE POSE: *We come now to a group of asans that are done on one leg at a time. These one-legged poses help to produce strong, one-pointed concentration. They also help to improve the blood circulation and to strengthen the ankles, knees and hips. This first asan is called the "Tree," for when one does this correctly, it makes the mind as steady as an oak.*

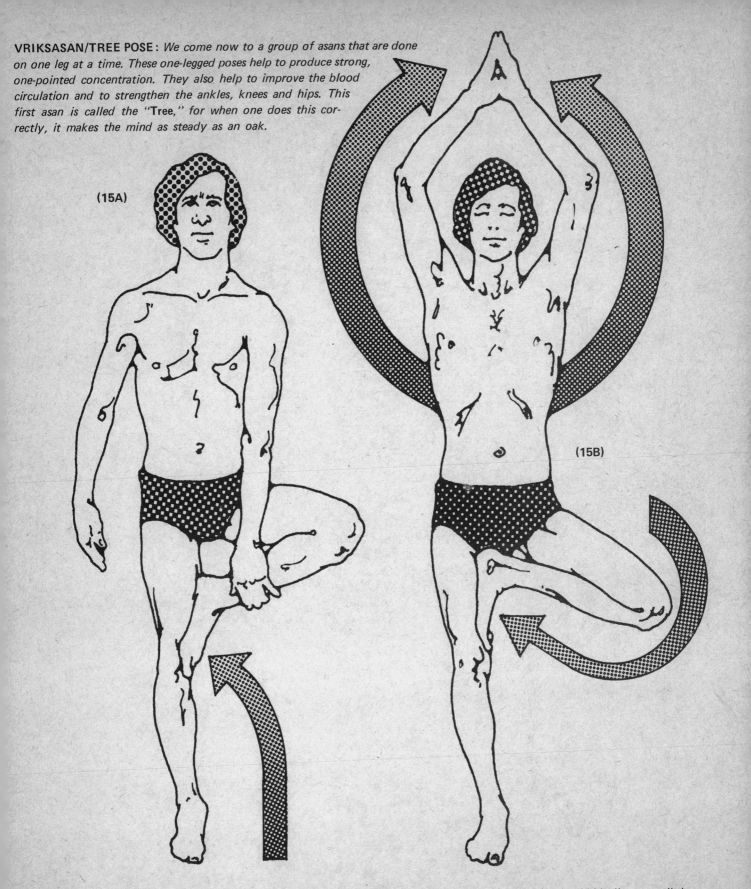

(15A)

(15B)

Begin by lifting the left foot and place it firmly on the inside of the right thigh (15A). The foot should ideally come all the way up on the thigh as in (15B). However, if your knees and thighs are too stiff, just bring the foot as high as you can. Once your foot is placed firmly on the thigh, fix the gaze on one spot without blinking. Now, slowly lift your hands in a gentle arc overhead. Place the palms together and push up slightly with the hands, straightening the arms (15B). Hold this position with gentle deep breathing as long as you can comfortably. When you become more sure of your balance try closing your eyes. Do this exercise once on each leg.

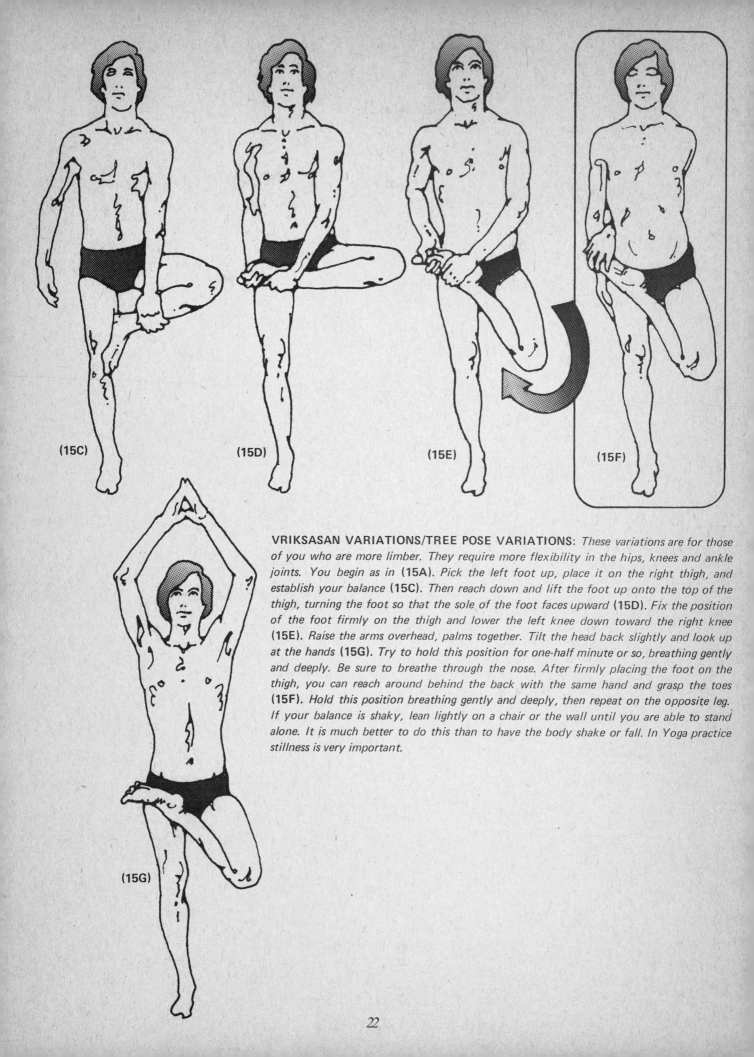

(15C)

(15D)

(15E)

(15F)

(15G)

VRIKSASAN VARIATIONS/TREE POSE VARIATIONS: *These variations are for those of you who are more limber. They require more flexibility in the hips, knees and ankle joints. You begin as in* **(15A)**. *Pick the left foot up, place it on the right thigh, and establish your balance* **(15C)**. *Then reach down and lift the foot up onto the top of the thigh, turning the foot so that the sole of the foot faces upward* **(15D)**. *Fix the position of the foot firmly on the thigh and lower the left knee down toward the right knee* **(15E)**. *Raise the arms overhead, palms together. Tilt the head back slightly and look up at the hands* **(15G)**. *Try to hold this position for one-half minute or so, breathing gently and deeply. Be sure to breathe through the nose. After firmly placing the foot on the thigh, you can reach around behind the back with the same hand and grasp the toes* **(15F)**. *Hold this position breathing gently and deeply, then repeat on the opposite leg. If your balance is shaky, lean lightly on a chair or the wall until you are able to stand alone. It is much better to do this than to have the body shake or fall. In Yoga practice stillness is very important.*

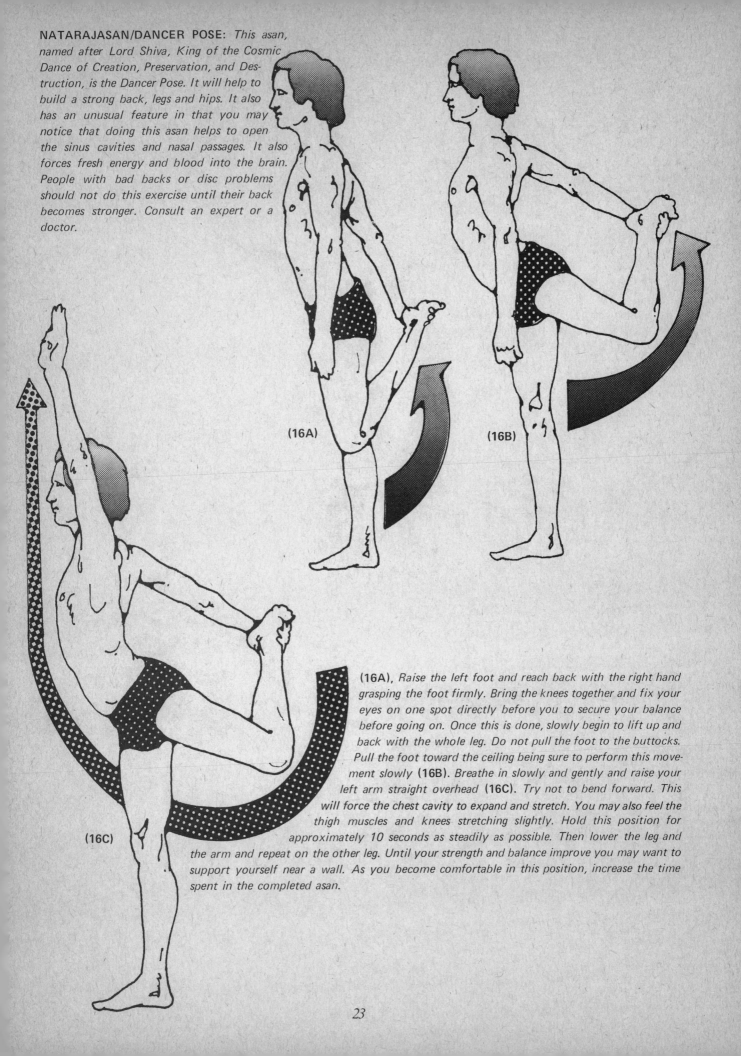

NATARAJASAN/DANCER POSE: *This asan, named after Lord Shiva, King of the Cosmic Dance of Creation, Preservation, and Destruction, is the Dancer Pose. It will help to build a strong back, legs and hips. It also has an unusual feature in that you may notice that doing this asan helps to open the sinus cavities and nasal passages. It also forces fresh energy and blood into the brain. People with bad backs or disc problems should not do this exercise until their back becomes stronger. Consult an expert or a doctor.*

(16A)

(16B)

(16C)

(16A), *Raise the left foot and reach back with the right hand grasping the foot firmly. Bring the knees together and fix your eyes on one spot directly before you to secure your balance before going on. Once this is done, slowly begin to lift up and back with the whole leg. Do not pull the foot to the buttocks. Pull the foot toward the ceiling being sure to perform this movement slowly* **(16B)**. *Breathe in slowly and gently and raise your left arm straight overhead* **(16C)**. *Try not to bend forward. This will force the chest cavity to expand and stretch. You may also feel the thigh muscles and knees stretching slightly. Hold this position for approximately 10 seconds as steadily as possible. Then lower the leg and the arm and repeat on the other leg. Until your strength and balance improve you may want to support yourself near a wall. As you become comfortable in this position, increase the time spent in the completed asan.*

23

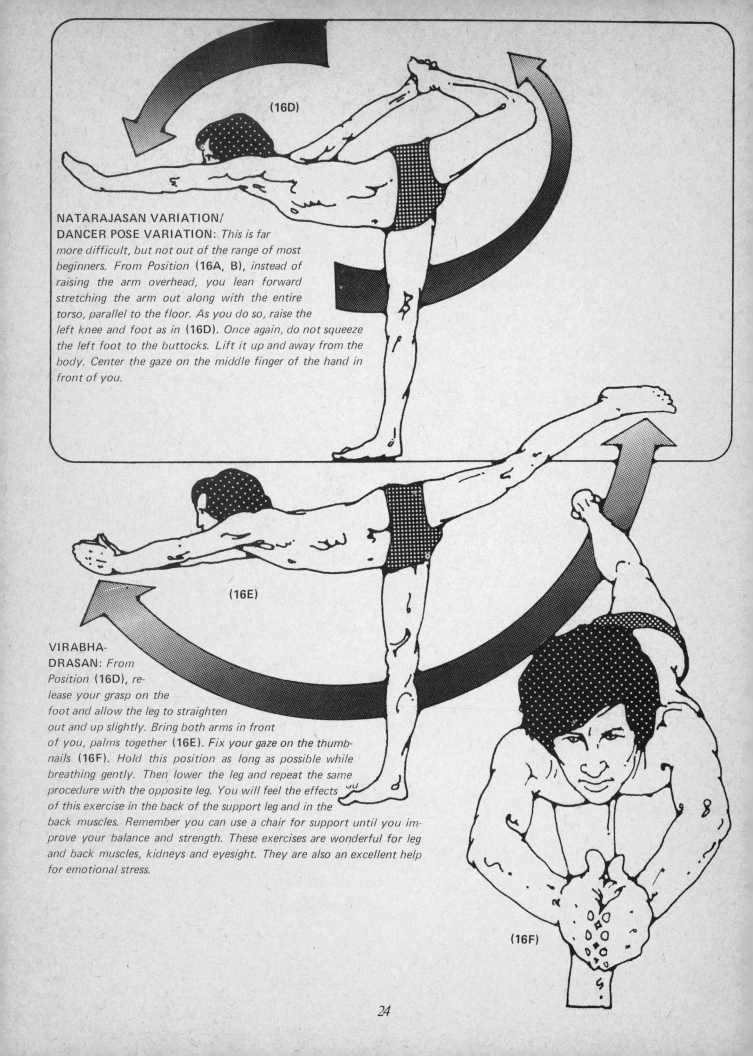

(16D)

**NATARAJASAN VARIATION/
DANCER POSE VARIATION:** *This is far
more difficult, but not out of the range of most
beginners. From Position* **(16A, B)**, *instead of
raising the arm overhead, you lean forward
stretching the arm out along with the entire
torso, parallel to the floor. As you do so, raise the
left knee and foot as in* **(16D)**. *Once again, do not squeeze
the left foot to the buttocks. Lift it up and away from the
body. Center the gaze on the middle finger of the hand in
front of you.*

(16E)

**VIRABHA-
DRASAN:** *From
Position* **(16D)**, *re-
lease your grasp on the
foot and allow the leg to straighten
out and up slightly. Bring both arms in front
of you, palms together* **(16E)**. *Fix your gaze on the thumb-
nails* **(16F)**. *Hold this position as long as possible while
breathing gently. Then lower the leg and repeat the same
procedure with the opposite leg. You will feel the effects
of this exercise in the back of the support leg and in the
back muscles. Remember you can use a chair for support until you improve your balance and strength. These exercises are wonderful for leg
and back muscles, kidneys and eyesight. They are also an excellent help
for emotional stress.*

(16F)

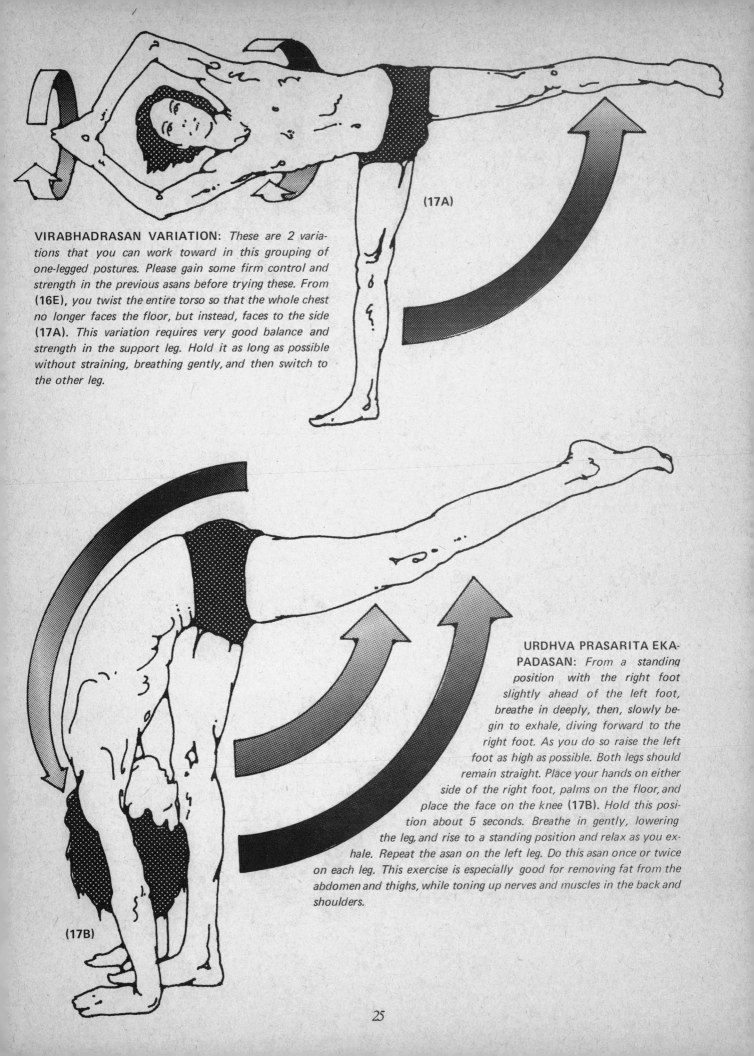

VIRABHADRASAN VARIATION: *These are 2 variations that you can work toward in this grouping of one-legged postures. Please gain some firm control and strength in the previous asans before trying these. From (16E), you twist the entire torso so that the whole chest no longer faces the floor, but instead, faces to the side (17A). This variation requires very good balance and strength in the support leg. Hold it as long as possible without straining, breathing gently, and then switch to the other leg.*

(17A)

URDHVA PRASARITA EKA-PADASAN: *From a standing position with the right foot slightly ahead of the left foot, breathe in deeply, then, slowly begin to exhale, diving forward to the right foot. As you do so raise the left foot as high as possible. Both legs should remain straight. Place your hands on either side of the right foot, palms on the floor, and place the face on the knee (17B). Hold this position about 5 seconds. Breathe in gently, lowering the leg, and rise to a standing position and relax as you exhale. Repeat the asan on the left leg. Do this asan once or twice on each leg. This exercise is especially good for removing fat from the abdomen and thighs, while toning up nerves and muscles in the back and shoulders.*

(17B)

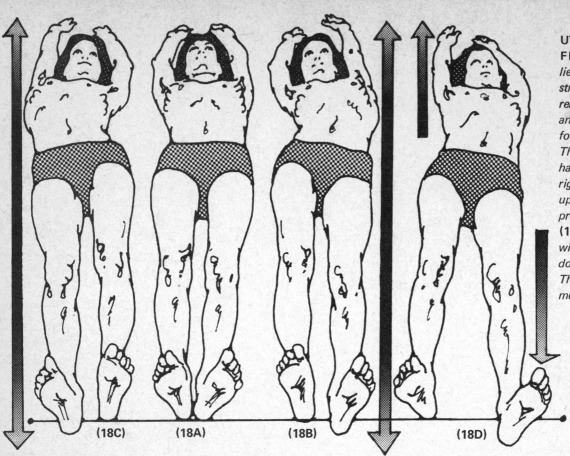

UTTIHITASAN / INTENSE FLOOR STRETCH: (18A), lie flat on the floor, arms straight overhead. (18B), reach up with the left hand and press down with the left foot keeping the foot flexed. Then, reach up with the right hand and press down with the right foot (18C). Now, reach up with the right hand and press down with the left foot (18D), and then reach up with the right hand and press down with the left foot. This exercise is a swivel movement of the hips.

(18C)   (18A)   (18B)   (18D)

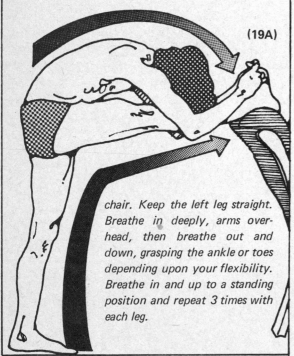

PADAHASTHAN VARIATION: *This stretch* (19A), *requires a chair or window ledge. Pick up your right foot and place it on the back of the*

(19A)

chair. Keep the left leg straight. Breathe in deeply, arms overhead, then breathe out and down, grasping the ankle or toes depending upon your flexibility. Breathe in and up to a standing position and repeat 3 times with each leg.

RAMA'S EASY POSE (3): *Nearly anyone can do this simple exercise, even invalids and bed-patients.* (20A), *make a fist with the hands, flex the toes and feet back toward the chest. Spread the fingers open and apart as far as possible and flex the toes and feet forward* (20B). *This is very easy, but effective in loosening the muscles and nerves in the legs. This will help keep good circulation in the legs and back. It is helpful for varicose veins or bedsores and removes fat from thighs and hips.*

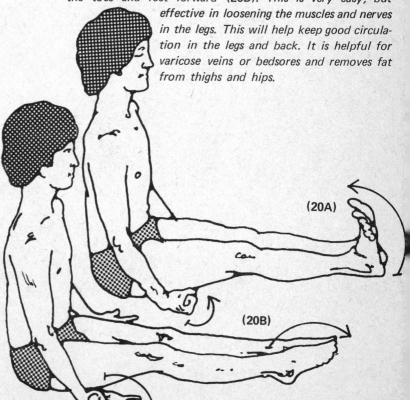

(20A)

(20B)

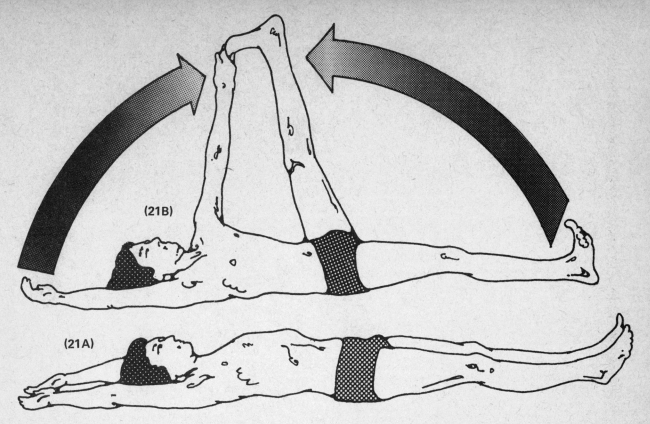

SUPTAPADANGUSTHASAN: *Lie flat on your back with your arms extended overhead* **(21A)**. *Breathe in and raise the left leg as you reach up with the left arm. Grasp the toes and hold this position keeping both legs as straight as possible* **(21B)**. *Notice that the right leg remains straight on the floor. Even if you can't grab the toes as in* **(21B)**, *try to reach them. With practice you will. Breathe out and lower the leg slowly to the floor. Repeat three times on each leg.*

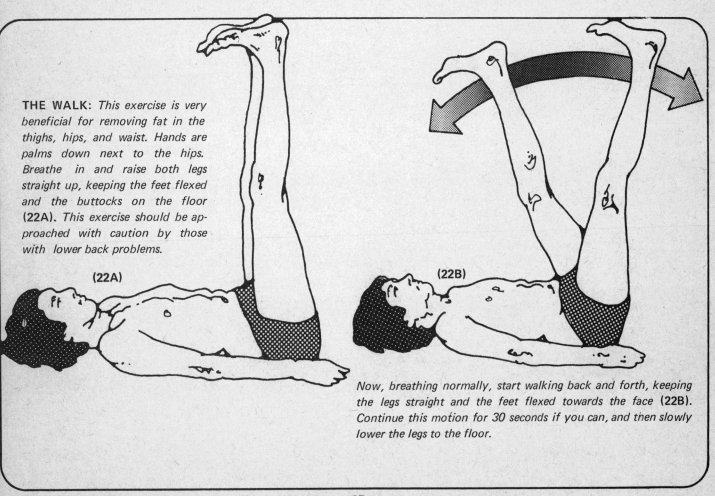

THE WALK: *This exercise is very beneficial for removing fat in the thighs, hips, and waist. Hands are palms down next to the hips. Breathe in and raise both legs straight up, keeping the feet flexed and the buttocks on the floor* **(22A)**. *This exercise should be approached with caution by those with lower back problems.*

Now, breathing normally, start walking back and forth, keeping the legs straight and the feet flexed towards the face **(22B)**. *Continue this motion for 30 seconds if you can, and then slowly lower the legs to the floor.*

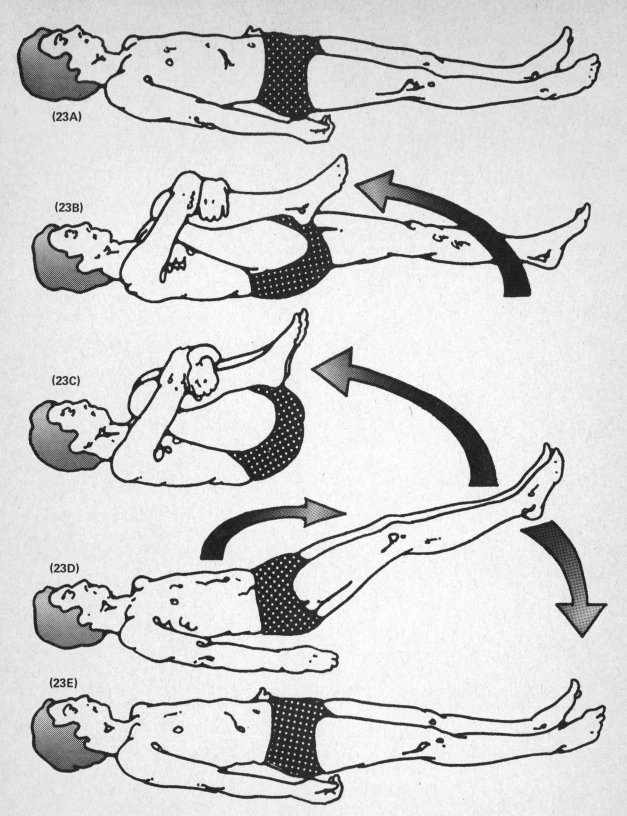

(23A)

(23B)

(23C)

(23D)

(23E)

PAVANAMUKTASAN/KNEE SQUEEZE: *Lie flat on your back with your arms to the sides, palms up* **(23A)**. *Begin to breathe in and raise the right knee to the chest. Fill your lungs and reach around the knee with your arms. Hold the breath and squeeze the knee to the chest for 5 seconds* **(23B)**. *Exhale slowly and straighten the leg. Repeat 1 or 2 times with each leg. In* **(23C)**, *a variation of this, you breathe in fully, raising both legs to the chest. Reach around the legs with the arms, hold the breath and squeeze the knees to the chest for 5 seconds. Then lower the legs* **(23D)**. *Exhale slowly and keep the legs straight all the way to the floor and relax* **(23E)**. *Repeat 3 times. This asan can also be done starting from Position* **(21A)**, *and returning to* **(21A)**, *as you relax. This asan helps to remove excess gas and distension of the bowels, relieves heartburn and increases blood circulation to the head. It also helps cure impotency.*

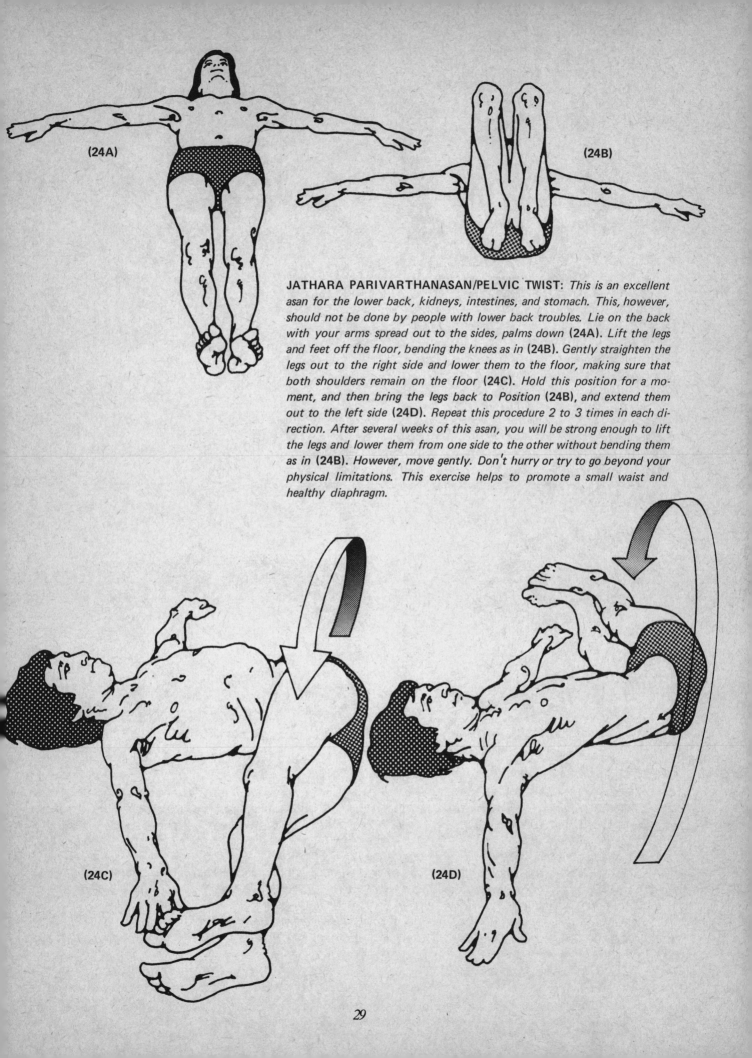

(24A)

(24B)

JATHARA PARIVARTHANASAN/PELVIC TWIST: *This is an excellent asan for the lower back, kidneys, intestines, and stomach. This, however, should not be done by people with lower back troubles. Lie on the back with your arms spread out to the sides, palms down* **(24A)**. *Lift the legs and feet off the floor, bending the knees as in* **(24B)**. *Gently straighten the legs out to the right side and lower them to the floor, making sure that both shoulders remain on the floor* **(24C)**. *Hold this position for a moment, and then bring the legs back to Position* **(24B)**, *and extend them out to the left side* **(24D)**. *Repeat this procedure 2 to 3 times in each direction. After several weeks of this asan, you will be strong enough to lift the legs and lower them from one side to the other without bending them as in* **(24B)**. *However, move gently. Don't hurry or try to go beyond your physical limitations. This exercise helps to promote a small waist and healthy diaphragm.*

(24C)

(24D)

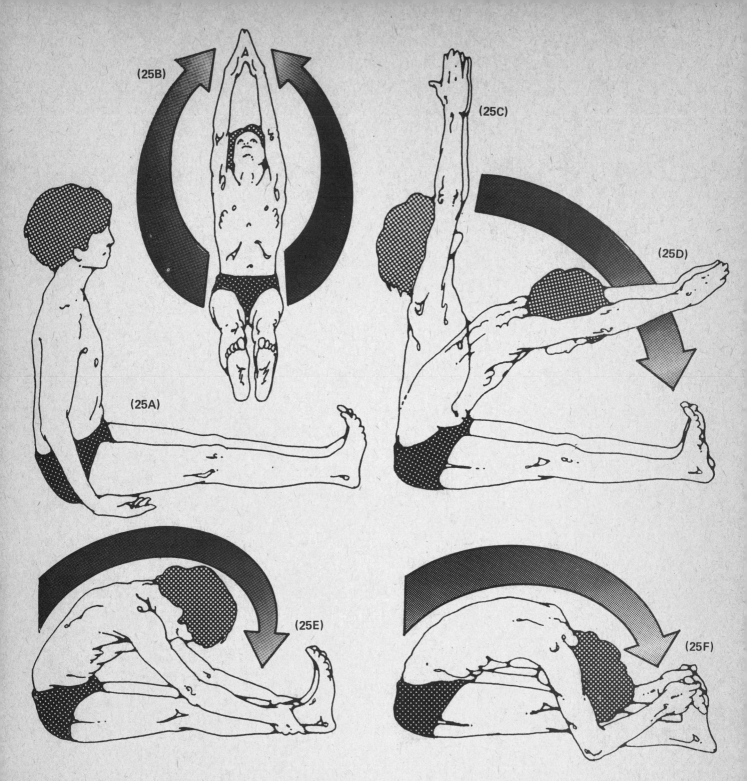

(25B)

(25C)

(25D)

(25A)

(25E)

(25F)

PASCHIMOTTANASAN/SEATED SUN POSE: *Start with both legs straight out in front of you, back straight and the arms to the side* **(25A)**. *As in the Standing Padahasthanasan, breathe in slowly and deeply through your nose, raising your arms in a large, circular motion over your head* **(25B)**. *This is to insure correct functioning of the lungs. Look up at the fingers for just a moment, then begin to breathe out slowly through the nose. As you do so, bend from the hips, keeping the knees flat on the floor and the legs straight with the feet flexed toward the face* **(25C, D)**. *By now you should have exhaled the air from the lungs* **(25E)**, *and for most beginners, this will be as far as you will be able to bend and stretch, so grasp the ankles firmly and pull gently trying to bring the head to the knees. After holding this Position* **(25E)**, *for 2 to 5 seconds, release the grip on the ankles, begin to breathe in gently, and come up slowly, as you fill the lungs, to Position* **(25B)**. *Relax and breathe out to* **(25A)**. *Repeat this pose 3 times. After you have practiced this asan for several weeks, you will notice that your legs and back are becoming supple and strong. Press on gently and in a short time you will be doing the completed asan with the elbows touching the floor, head between the knees, fingers grasping the toes and a full, rejuvenating stretch to the spine and legs* **(25F, G)**.

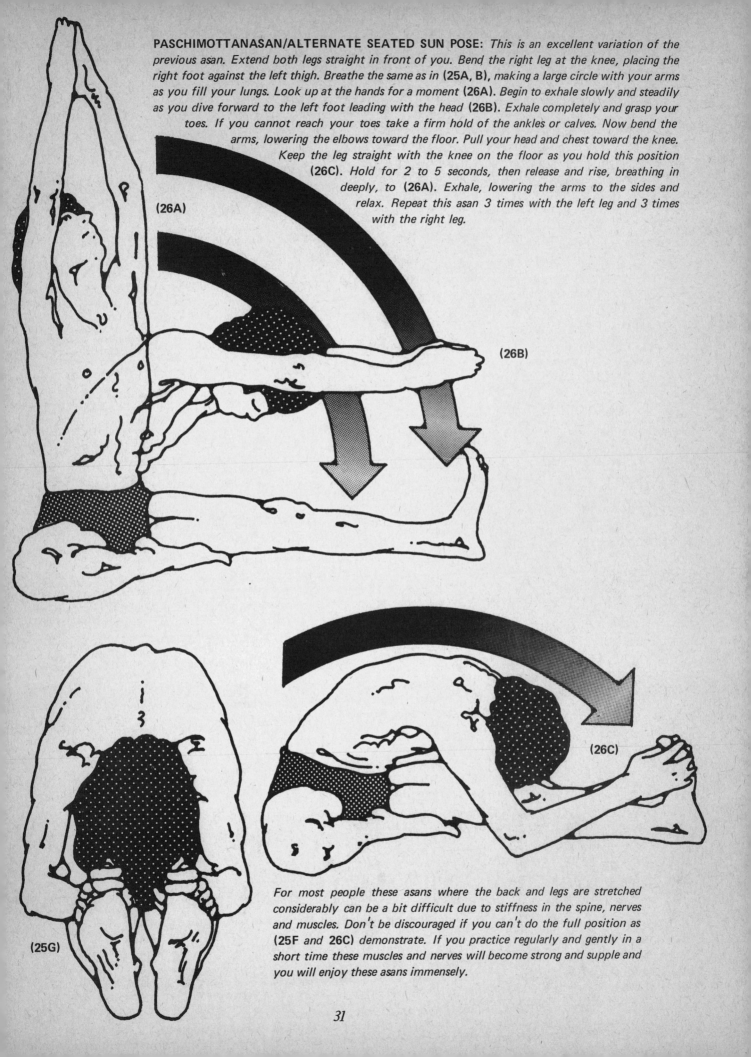

PASCHIMOTTANASAN/ALTERNATE SEATED SUN POSE: *This is an excellent variation of the previous asan. Extend both legs straight in front of you. Bend the right leg at the knee, placing the right foot against the left thigh. Breathe the same as in* (25A, B), *making a large circle with your arms as you fill your lungs. Look up at the hands for a moment* (26A). *Begin to exhale slowly and steadily as you dive forward to the left foot leading with the head* (26B). *Exhale completely and grasp your toes. If you cannot reach your toes take a firm hold of the ankles or calves. Now bend the arms, lowering the elbows toward the floor. Pull your head and chest toward the knee. Keep the leg straight with the knee on the floor as you hold this position* (26C). *Hold for 2 to 5 seconds, then release and rise, breathing in deeply, to* (26A). *Exhale, lowering the arms to the sides and relax. Repeat this asan 3 times with the left leg and 3 times with the right leg.*

(26A)

(26B)

(25G)

(26C)

For most people these asans where the back and legs are stretched considerably can be a bit difficult due to stiffness in the spine, nerves and muscles. Don't be discouraged if you can't do the full position as (25F *and* 26C) *demonstrate. If you practice regularly and gently in a short time these muscles and nerves will become strong and supple and you will enjoy these asans immensely.*

31

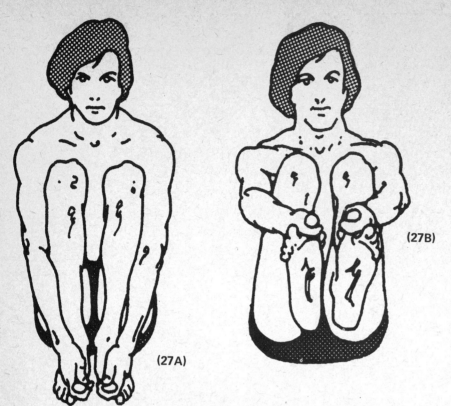

(27B)

(27A)

PASCHIMOTTANASAN VARIATION: *This is an exercise you will enjoy trying. Even if you can't do it quite as well as is shown here, do not be discouraged. With practice you will be doing it perfectly. The most important thing is to retain balance.* (**27A**), *sit on the buttocks and pull the knees to the chest. Reach around the legs and grab the big toes or the feet. Now, sit back and balance on your buttocks holding the toes or feet with the knees bent* (**27B, C**). *Next, try, to straighten the legs fully and, if you can, pull the head to the knees. Hold this position breathing steadily* (**27D**). *This asan builds strength in the legs, abdomen and back. This exercise will also help cure impotency and help to develop and maintain good mental stability.*

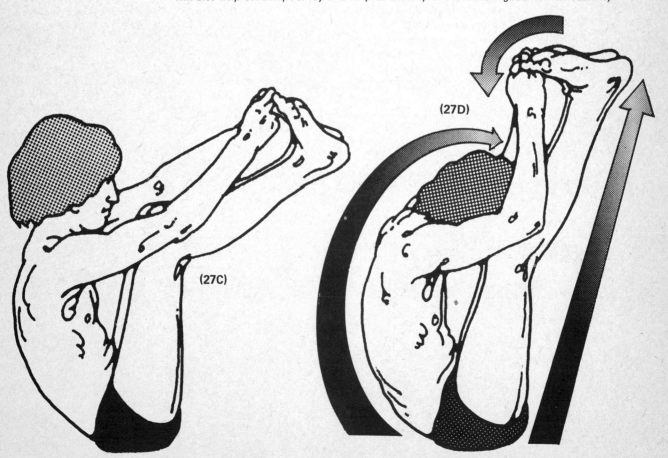

(27D)

(27C)

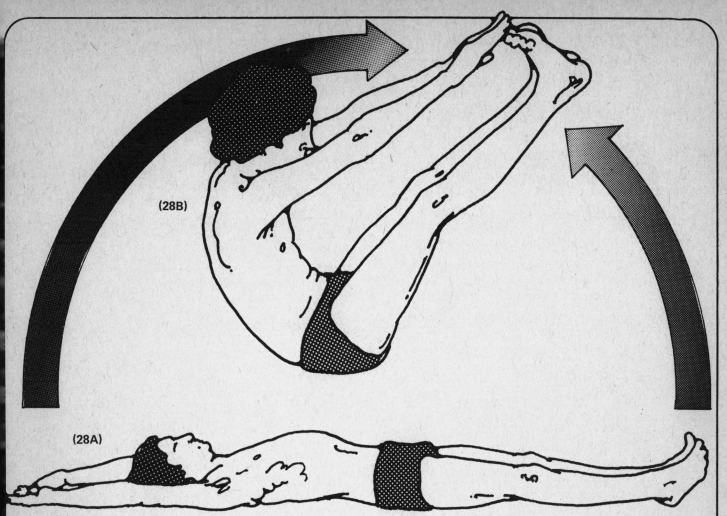

PADANGUSTHASAN/SPINE BALANCE: *This is more challenging than* **(27).** *Lie flat on the back with the arms extended overhead* **(28A).** *Breathe in, raising the arms and legs simultaneously. Balancing on the lower spine, reach up and rest the hands on top of the toes* **(28B).** *Do not grab them. Hold this position with your lungs filled for several seconds, then exhale as you lower the arms over the head and lower the legs to the floor.*

MATSYASAN/THE EASY FISH: *This is the beginning fish posture* **(29A).** *Lie flat on the back and slide the hands just under the thighs. Now use the arms and back muscles to lift your body, from the waist up, off the floor. Now arch the back and neck so that the top of the head rests on the floor. Keep the teeth and lips together and jut the lower jaw forward. Open the eyes and look at the floor breathing deeply and steadily. Hold this position for 10 to 15 seconds, then straighten the spine as you lower to the floor and relax. This asan removes facial lines and neck wrinkles. It also makes the eyes clear and bright, improves the voice and cures diseases of the throat.*

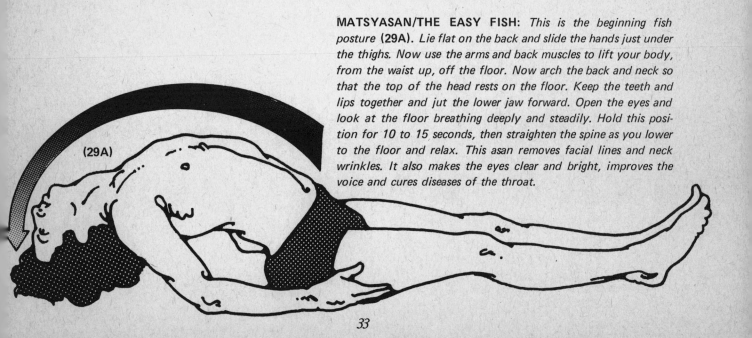

ROWBOAT: *This is an exercise we use in our classes to limber the legs and back.* **(30A)**, *the feet and legs should be spread wide apart and the bottoms of your feet placed on the bottoms of your partner's feet. Reach over and lock wrists with your partner. Now, pull gently on your partner's arms as you lean back slightly. This will pull your partner toward you. Your partner should try to put his head on the floor* **(30B)**. *Release your pull, allowing him to come up and then repeat the process 2 to 3 times. Then your partner pulls you. Do not jerk or pull violently.*

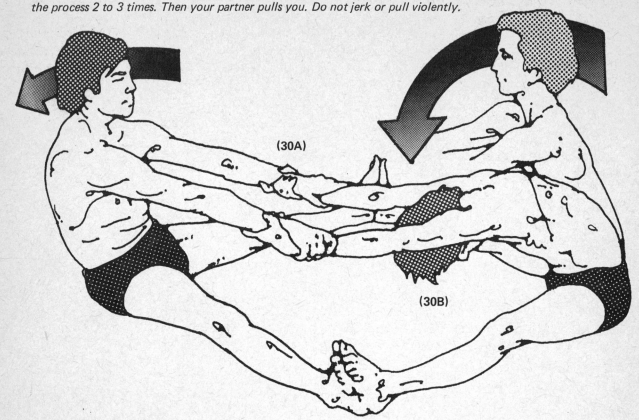

(30A)

(30B)

VIRASAN VARIATION/HERO POSE VARIATION: *This is an excellent pose for women because it exercises the lower pelvic region including the kidneys, lower back, hips, thighs and the ovarian system. Sit on the feet with your arms overhead, one hand on top of the other* **(31A)**. *Breathing deeply while rising off the feet several inches, begin to exhale and slide to the right. Finish exhaling as you sit down* **(31B)**. *Try to keep the knees on the floor as you move. Breathe in and lift up and over to* **(31A)**. *Then exhale as you lower to the left side as in* **(31C)**. *This process should be repeated 3 times to the left and 3 times to the right, returning to the center position* **(31A)** *as you finish.*

(31B)

(31A)

(31C)

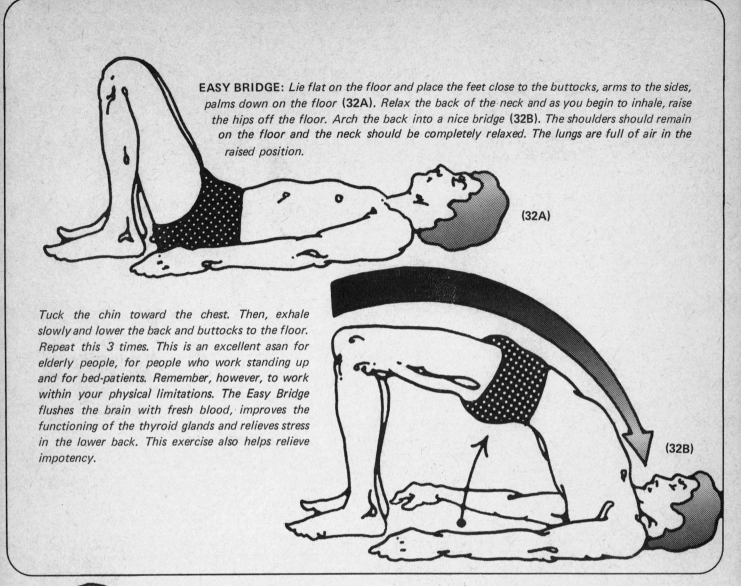

EASY BRIDGE: *Lie flat on the floor and place the feet close to the buttocks, arms to the sides, palms down on the floor* **(32A)**. *Relax the back of the neck and as you begin to inhale, raise the hips off the floor. Arch the back into a nice bridge* **(32B)**. *The shoulders should remain on the floor and the neck should be completely relaxed. The lungs are full of air in the raised position.*

(32A)

Tuck the chin toward the chest. Then, exhale slowly and lower the back and buttocks to the floor. Repeat this 3 times. This is an excellent asan for elderly people, for people who work standing up and for bed-patients. Remember, however, to work within your physical limitations. The Easy Bridge flushes the brain with fresh blood, improves the functioning of the thyroid glands and relieves stress in the lower back. This exercise also helps relieve impotency.

(32B)

VIRASAN VARIATION/HERO POSE VARIATION: *This is one of the easiest and most beneficial postures for beginners. It relieves stress in the back, neck and shoulders. It improves blood circulation and relieves stress, headaches, eye disease, and makes the mind bright and alert. Sit on the feet with the toes touching and the heels separated to the sides* **(33A)**. *Place your hands, palms up, next to the feet. Exhale and fold in half, resting the head on the floor* **(33B)**. *Completely relax the shoulders and neck and breathe normally. Hold this position as long as is comfortable. You may notice a slight pounding of the blood in the arteries of the neck. This is normal because the head is below the heart enabling the blood to flow easily. The pounding should ease in 15 to 30 seconds. The knees should remain together throughout this asan.*

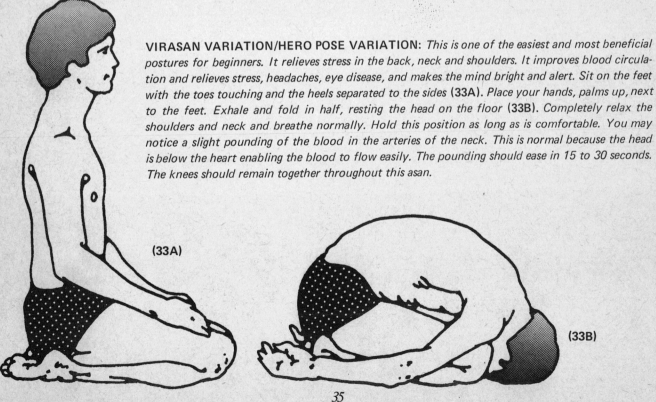

(33A)

(33B)

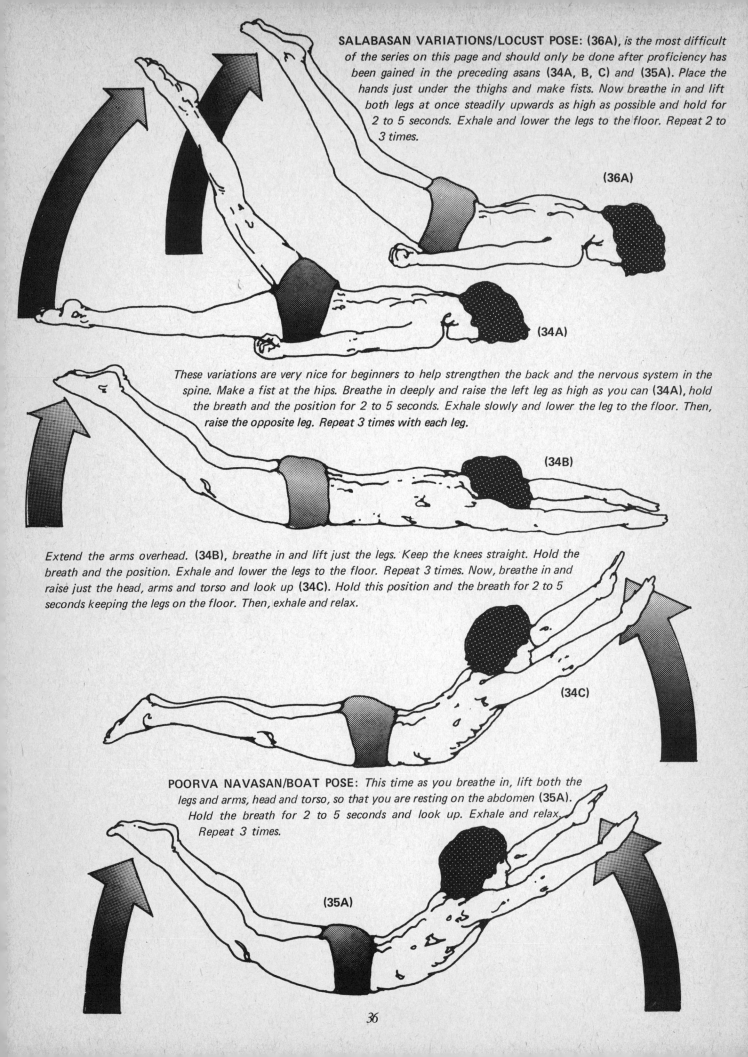

SALABASAN VARIATIONS/LOCUST POSE: (36A), *is the most difficult of the series on this page and should only be done after proficiency has been gained in the preceding asans (34A, B, C) and (35A). Place the hands just under the thighs and make fists. Now breathe in and lift both legs at once steadily upwards as high as possible and hold for 2 to 5 seconds. Exhale and lower the legs to the floor. Repeat 2 to 3 times.*

(36A)

(34A)

These variations are very nice for beginners to help strengthen the back and the nervous system in the spine. Make a fist at the hips. Breathe in deeply and raise the left leg as high as you can (34A), hold the breath and the position for 2 to 5 seconds. Exhale slowly and lower the leg to the floor. Then, raise the opposite leg. Repeat 3 times with each leg.

(34B)

Extend the arms overhead. (34B), breathe in and lift just the legs. Keep the knees straight. Hold the breath and the position. Exhale and lower the legs to the floor. Repeat 3 times. Now, breathe in and raise just the head, arms and torso and look up (34C). Hold this position and the breath for 2 to 5 seconds keeping the legs on the floor. Then, exhale and relax.

(34C)

POORVA NAVASAN/BOAT POSE: *This time as you breathe in, lift both the legs and arms, head and torso, so that you are resting on the abdomen (35A). Hold the breath for 2 to 5 seconds and look up. Exhale and relax. Repeat 3 times.*

(35A)

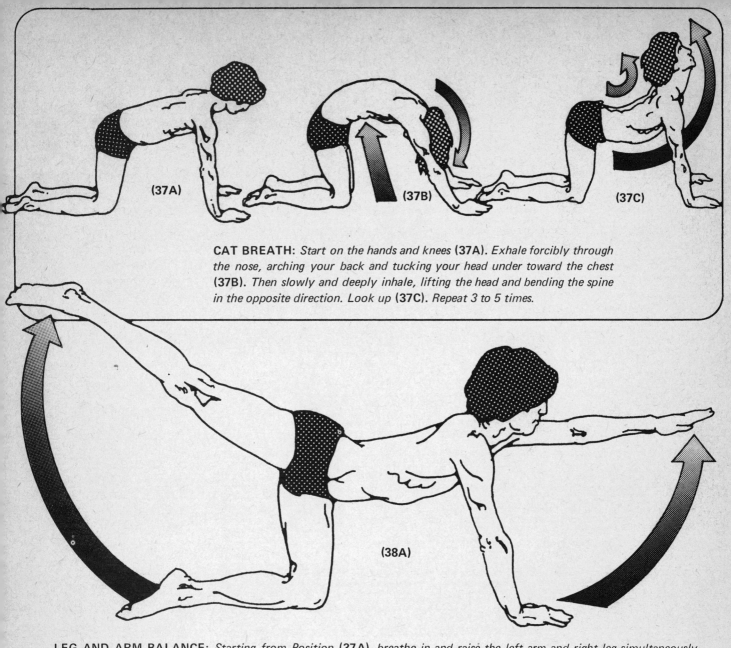

CAT BREATH: *Start on the hands and knees (37A). Exhale forcibly through the nose, arching your back and tucking your head under toward the chest (37B). Then slowly and deeply inhale, lifting the head and bending the spine in the opposite direction. Look up (37C). Repeat 3 to 5 times.*

(37A)

(37B)

(37C)

(38A)

LEG AND ARM BALANCE: *Starting from Position (37A), breathe in and raise the left arm and right leg simultaneously (38A). Hold this position for 5 to 10 seconds, breathing gently. Lower the right leg and left arm and then raise the left leg and right arm. Repeat this process 3 times. In a variation (38B), the breathing is the same except that you raise both the right leg and right arm simultaneously. Hold this position without leaning to the side. Repeat this exercise 2 or 3 times on each side of the body.*

(38B)

37

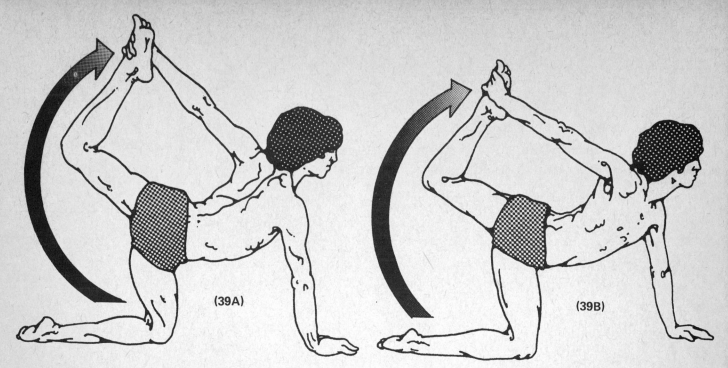

DHANURASAN VARIATION/BOW POSTURE: *Starting from Position* **(37A)**, *reach back and grasp the left foot with the left hand. Raise the foot and leg up as high as you can* **(39A)**, *and hold this position for several seconds. Then, lower the leg to the floor and repeat on the opposite side. Now, reach back with the right hand and grasp the left foot. Raise the foot and knee as high as you can* **(39B)**, *and hold this position for several seconds.*

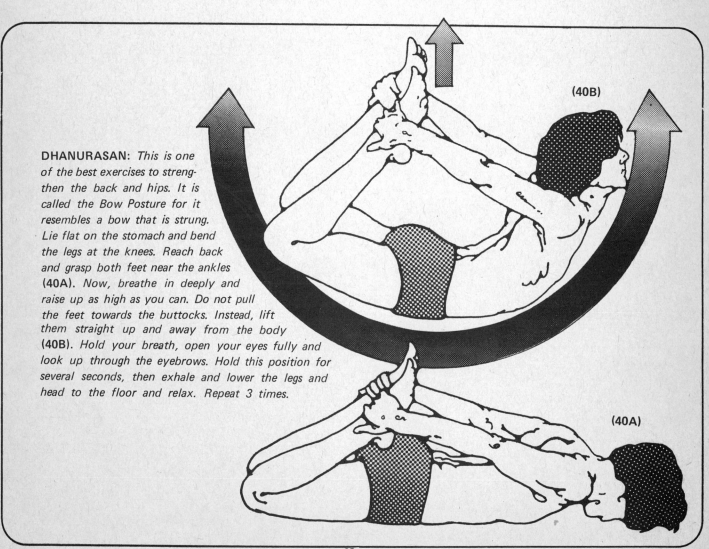

DHANURASAN: *This is one of the best exercises to strengthen the back and hips. It is called the Bow Posture for it resembles a bow that is strung. Lie flat on the stomach and bend the legs at the knees. Reach back and grasp both feet near the ankles* **(40A)**. *Now, breathe in deeply and raise up as high as you can. Do not pull the feet towards the buttocks. Instead, lift them straight up and away from the body* **(40B)**. *Hold your breath, open your eyes fully and look up through the eyebrows. Hold this position for several seconds, then exhale and lower the legs and head to the floor and relax. Repeat 3 times.*

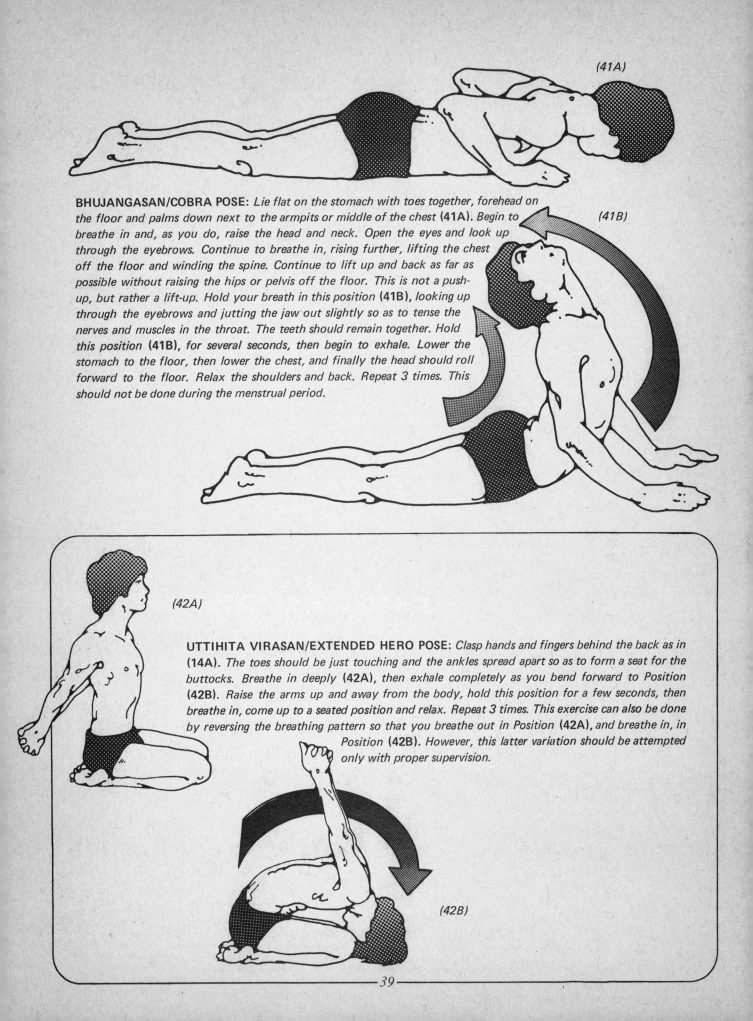

BHUJANGASAN/COBRA POSE: *Lie flat on the stomach with toes together, forehead on the floor and palms down next to the armpits or middle of the chest* **(41A)**. *Begin to breathe in and, as you do, raise the head and neck. Open the eyes and look up through the eyebrows. Continue to breathe in, rising further, lifting the chest off the floor and winding the spine. Continue to lift up and back as far as possible without raising the hips or pelvis off the floor. This is not a push-up, but rather a lift-up. Hold your breath in this position* **(41B)**, *looking up through the eyebrows and jutting the jaw out slightly so as to tense the nerves and muscles in the throat. The teeth should remain together. Hold this position* **(41B)**, *for several seconds, then begin to exhale. Lower the stomach to the floor, then lower the chest, and finally the head should roll forward to the floor. Relax the shoulders and back. Repeat 3 times. This should not be done during the menstrual period.*

(41A)

(41B)

(42A)

UTTIHITA VIRASAN/EXTENDED HERO POSE: *Clasp hands and fingers behind the back as in* **(14A)**. *The toes should be just touching and the ankles spread apart so as to form a seat for the buttocks. Breathe in deeply* **(42A)**, *then exhale completely as you bend forward to Position* **(42B)**. *Raise the arms up and away from the body, hold this position for a few seconds, then breathe in, come up to a seated position and relax. Repeat 3 times. This exercise can also be done by reversing the breathing pattern so that you breathe out in Position* **(42A)**, *and breathe in, in Position* **(42B)**. *However, this latter variation should be attempted only with proper supervision.*

(42B)

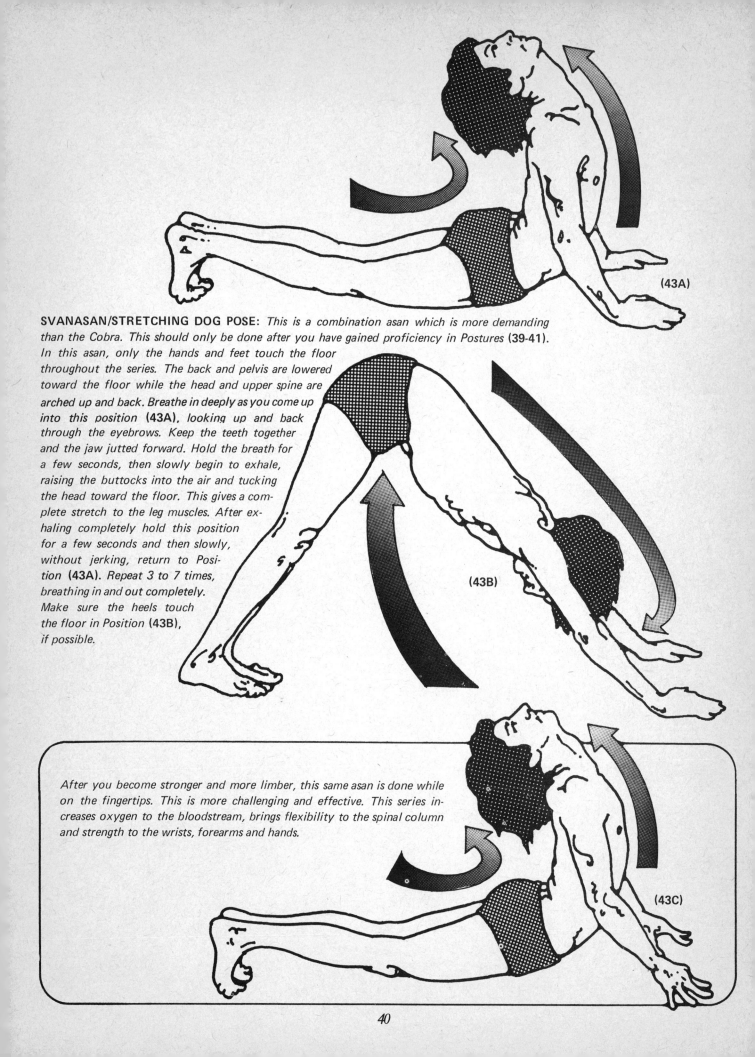

SVANASAN/STRETCHING DOG POSE: *This is a combination asan which is more demanding than the Cobra. This should only be done after you have gained proficiency in Postures (39-41). In this asan, only the hands and feet touch the floor throughout the series. The back and pelvis are lowered toward the floor while the head and upper spine are arched up and back. Breathe in deeply as you come up into this position (43A), looking up and back through the eyebrows. Keep the teeth together and the jaw jutted forward. Hold the breath for a few seconds, then slowly begin to exhale, raising the buttocks into the air and tucking the head toward the floor. This gives a complete stretch to the leg muscles. After exhaling completely hold this position for a few seconds and then slowly, without jerking, return to Position (43A). Repeat 3 to 7 times, breathing in and out completely. Make sure the heels touch the floor in Position (43B), if possible.*

(43A)

(43B)

After you become stronger and more limber, this same asan is done while on the fingertips. This is more challenging and effective. This series increases oxygen to the bloodstream, brings flexibility to the spinal column and strength to the wrists, forearms and hands.

(43C)

HANUMANASAN PREPARATION: *This is an effective preparation for more advanced asans. However, it should not be done by women during the menstrual period, nor by women who have had difficulties with displacement of the uterus. If done properly, this asan has a very beneficial effect on the reproductive organs both for men and women. It also elongates the muscles and tendons of the thighs and hips. Come to Position* **(44A).** *Notice that you should be on your fingertips with the left knee resting on the floor. Now, point the left foot so that the top of it is on the floor. Raise the left knee off the floor and arch the back up with your eyes open* **(44B).** *Breathe naturally and try to hold this position for several seconds. Then, lower the left knee back to the floor. Sit back slightly, straightening the right leg.*

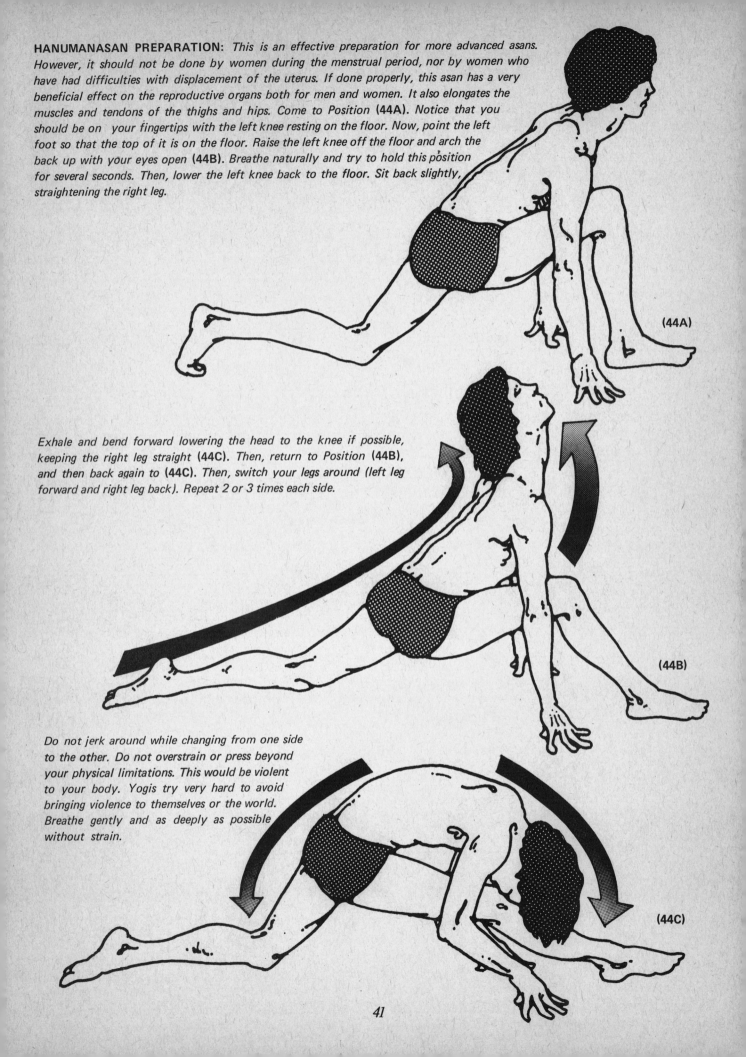

(44A)

Exhale and bend forward lowering the head to the knee if possible, keeping the right leg straight **(44C).** *Then, return to Position* **(44B),** *and then back again to* **(44C).** *Then, switch your legs around (left leg forward and right leg back). Repeat 2 or 3 times each side.*

(44B)

Do not jerk around while changing from one side to the other. Do not overstrain or press beyond your physical limitations. This would be violent to your body. Yogis try very hard to avoid bringing violence to themselves or the world. Breathe gently and as deeply as possible without strain.

(44C)

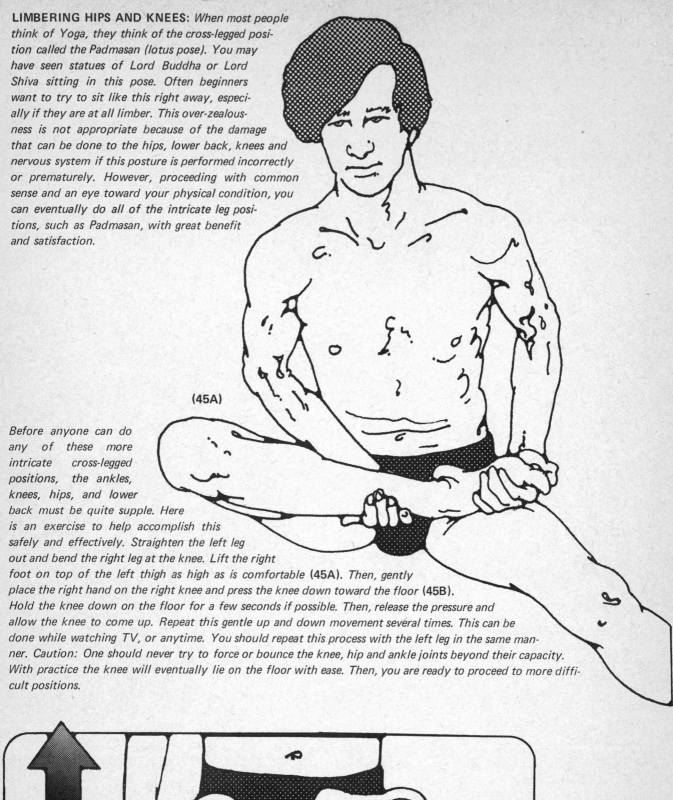

LIMBERING HIPS AND KNEES: *When most people think of Yoga, they think of the cross-legged position called the Padmasan (lotus pose). You may have seen statues of Lord Buddha or Lord Shiva sitting in this pose. Often beginners want to try to sit like this right away, especially if they are at all limber. This over-zealousness is not appropriate because of the damage that can be done to the hips, lower back, knees and nervous system if this posture is performed incorrectly or prematurely. However, proceeding with common sense and an eye toward your physical condition, you can eventually do all of the intricate leg positions, such as Padmasan, with great benefit and satisfaction.*

(45A)

Before anyone can do any of these more intricate cross-legged positions, the ankles, knees, hips, and lower back must be quite supple. Here is an exercise to help accomplish this safely and effectively. Straighten the left leg out and bend the right leg at the knee. Lift the right foot on top of the left thigh as high as is comfortable **(45A)**. *Then, gently place the right hand on the right knee and press the knee down toward the floor* **(45B)**. *Hold the knee down on the floor for a few seconds if possible. Then, release the pressure and allow the knee to come up. Repeat this gentle up and down movement several times. This can be done while watching TV, or anytime. You should repeat this process with the left leg in the same manner. Caution: One should never try to force or bounce the knee, hip and ankle joints beyond their capacity. With practice the knee will eventually lie on the floor with ease. Then, you are ready to proceed to more difficult positions.*

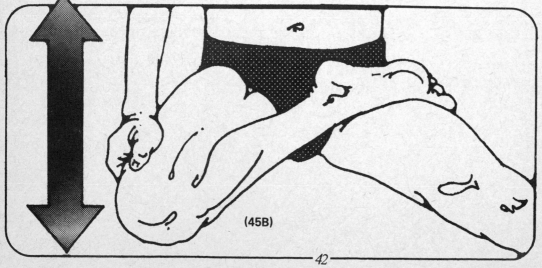

(45B)

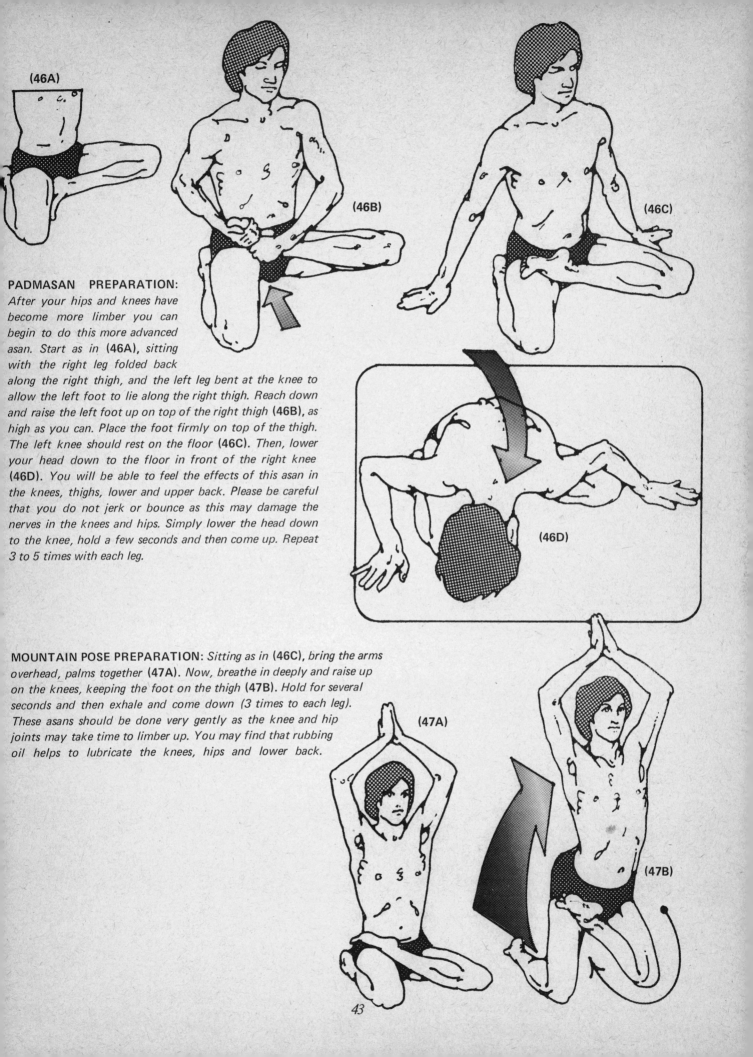

(46A)

(46B)

(46C)

PADMASAN PREPARATION:

After your hips and knees have become more limber you can begin to do this more advanced asan. Start as in (46A), sitting with the right leg folded back along the right thigh, and the left leg bent at the knee to allow the left foot to lie along the right thigh. Reach down and raise the left foot up on top of the right thigh (46B), as high as you can. Place the foot firmly on top of the thigh. The left knee should rest on the floor (46C). Then, lower your head down to the floor in front of the right knee (46D). You will be able to feel the effects of this asan in the knees, thighs, lower and upper back. Please be careful that you do not jerk or bounce as this may damage the nerves in the knees and hips. Simply lower the head down to the knee, hold a few seconds and then come up. Repeat 3 to 5 times with each leg.

(46D)

MOUNTAIN POSE PREPARATION:
Sitting as in (46C), bring the arms overhead, palms together (47A). Now, breathe in deeply and raise up on the knees, keeping the foot on the thigh (47B). Hold for several seconds and then exhale and come down (3 times to each leg). These asans should be done very gently as the knee and hip joints may take time to limber up. You may find that rubbing oil helps to lubricate the knees, hips and lower back.

(47A)

(47B)

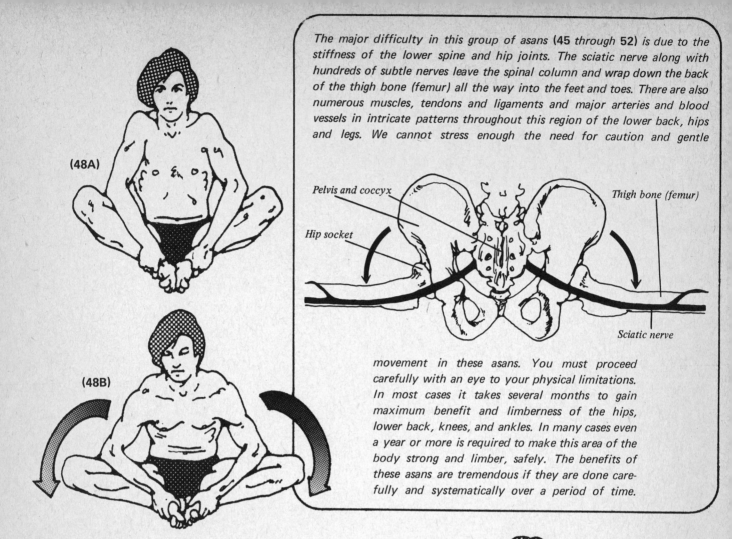

(48A)

(48B)

The major difficulty in this group of asans **(45 through 52)** is due to the stiffness of the lower spine and hip joints. The sciatic nerve along with hundreds of subtle nerves leave the spinal column and wrap down the back of the thigh bone (femur) all the way into the feet and toes. There are also numerous muscles, tendons and ligaments and major arteries and blood vessels in intricate patterns throughout this region of the lower back, hips and legs. We cannot stress enough the need for caution and gentle

Pelvis and coccyx

Hip socket

Thigh bone (femur)

Sciatic nerve

movement in these asans. You must proceed carefully with an eye to your physical limitations. In most cases it takes several months to gain maximum benefit and limberness of the hips, lower back, knees, and ankles. In many cases even a year or more is required to make this area of the body strong and limber, safely. The benefits of these asans are tremendous if they are done carefully and systematically over a period of time.

BHADRASAN/SHIVA'S THRONE: *Sit on the buttocks* **(48A)**, *and put the bottoms of the feet together, pulling them as close into the groin as possible. Grasp the ankles, placing your elbows on the thighs. Breathe in deeply, then exhale slowly and completely, pressing the thighs and knees down to the floor* **(48B)**. *Hold for several seconds and release. Then breathe in and relax. Repeat 3 times.*

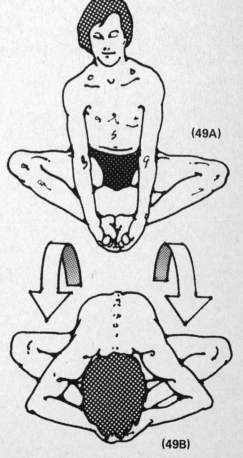

(49A)

(49B)

SHIVA SHAKTIASAN: *This exercise is a little more difficult. From Position* **(48A)**, *move the feet away from the groin approximately 12 inches. Interlock fingers under the toes. If possible, touch the forehead to the big toes and hold this position for a moment breathing normally. Then, come up and again lower to Position* **(49B)**. *Repeat 5 to 7 times.*

44

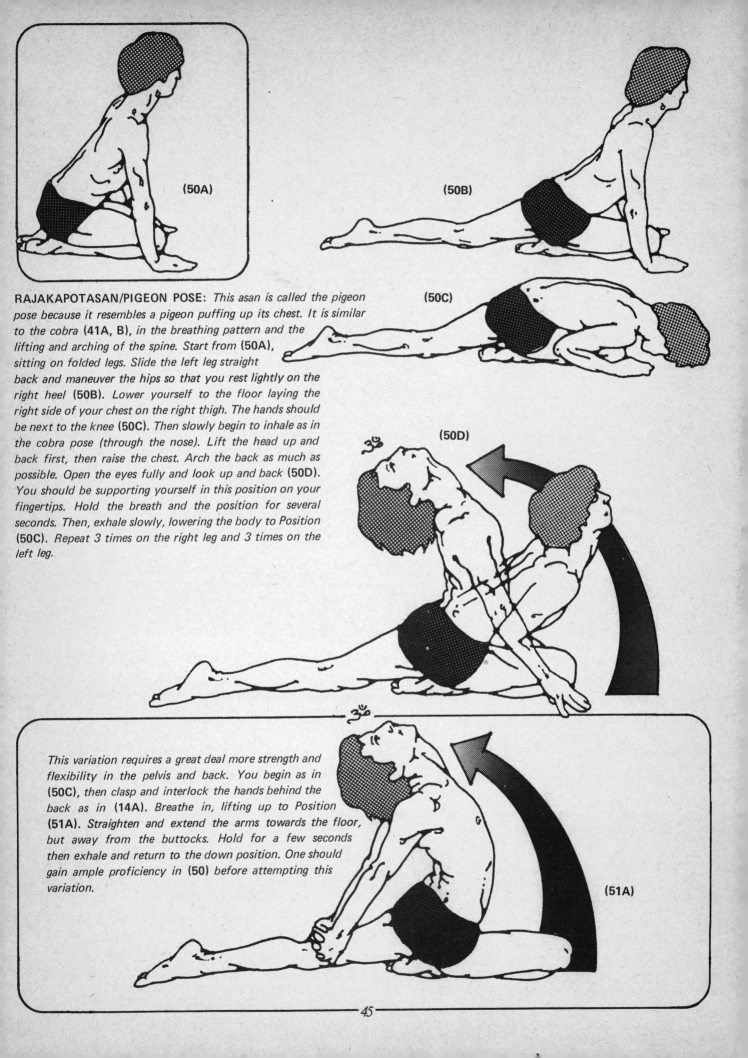

(50A)

(50B)

(50C)

RAJAKAPOTASAN/PIGEON POSE: *This asan is called the pigeon pose because it resembles a pigeon puffing up its chest. It is similar to the cobra (41A, B), in the breathing pattern and the lifting and arching of the spine. Start from (50A), sitting on folded legs. Slide the left leg straight back and maneuver the hips so that you rest lightly on the right heel (50B). Lower yourself to the floor laying the right side of your chest on the right thigh. The hands should be next to the knee (50C). Then slowly begin to inhale as in the cobra pose (through the nose). Lift the head up and back first, then raise the chest. Arch the back as much as possible. Open the eyes fully and look up and back (50D). You should be supporting yourself in this position on your fingertips. Hold the breath and the position for several seconds. Then, exhale slowly, lowering the body to Position (50C). Repeat 3 times on the right leg and 3 times on the left leg.*

(50D)

This variation requires a great deal more strength and flexibility in the pelvis and back. You begin as in (50C), then clasp and interlock the hands behind the back as in (14A). Breathe in, lifting up to Position (51A). Straighten and extend the arms towards the floor, but away from the buttocks. Hold for a few seconds then exhale and return to the down position. One should gain ample proficiency in (50) before attempting this variation.

(51A)

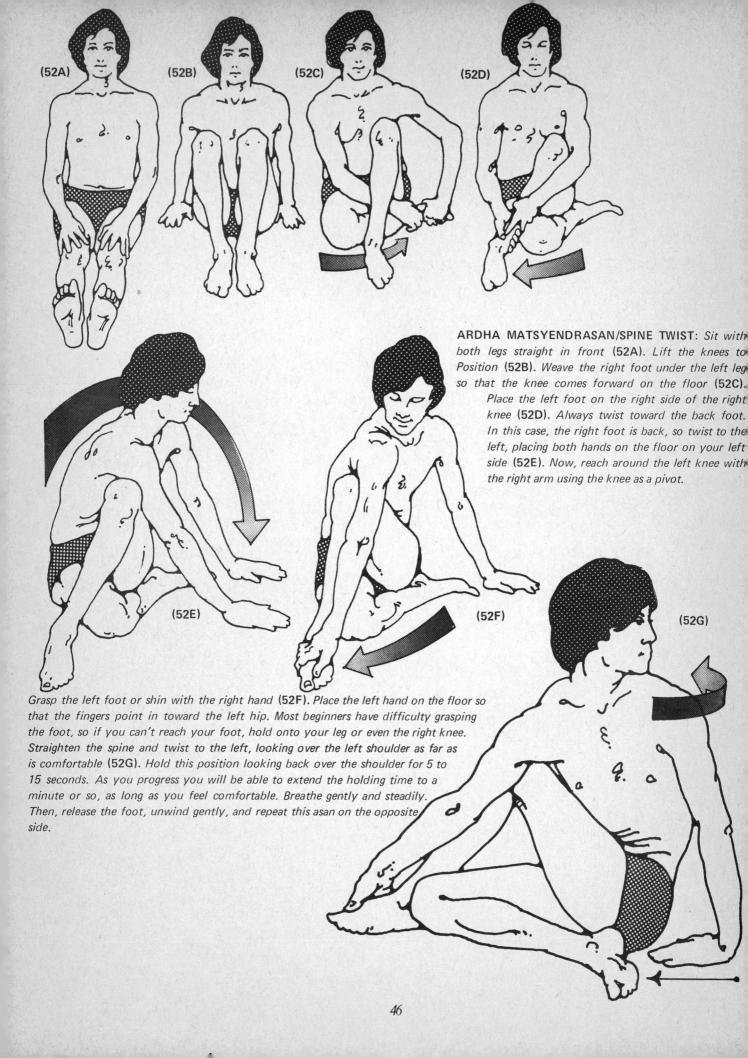

ARDHA MATSYENDRASAN/SPINE TWIST: *Sit with both legs straight in front (52A). Lift the knees to Position (52B). Weave the right foot under the left leg so that the knee comes forward on the floor (52C). Place the left foot on the right side of the right knee (52D). Always twist toward the back foot. In this case, the right foot is back, so twist to the left, placing both hands on the floor on your left side (52E). Now, reach around the left knee with the right arm using the knee as a pivot.*

Grasp the left foot or shin with the right hand (52F). Place the left hand on the floor so that the fingers point in toward the left hip. Most beginners have difficulty grasping the foot, so if you can't reach your foot, hold onto your leg or even the right knee. Straighten the spine and twist to the left, looking over the left shoulder as far as is comfortable (52G). Hold this position looking back over the shoulder for 5 to 15 seconds. As you progress you will be able to extend the holding time to a minute or so, as long as you feel comfortable. Breathe gently and steadily. Then, release the foot, unwind gently, and repeat this asan on the opposite side.

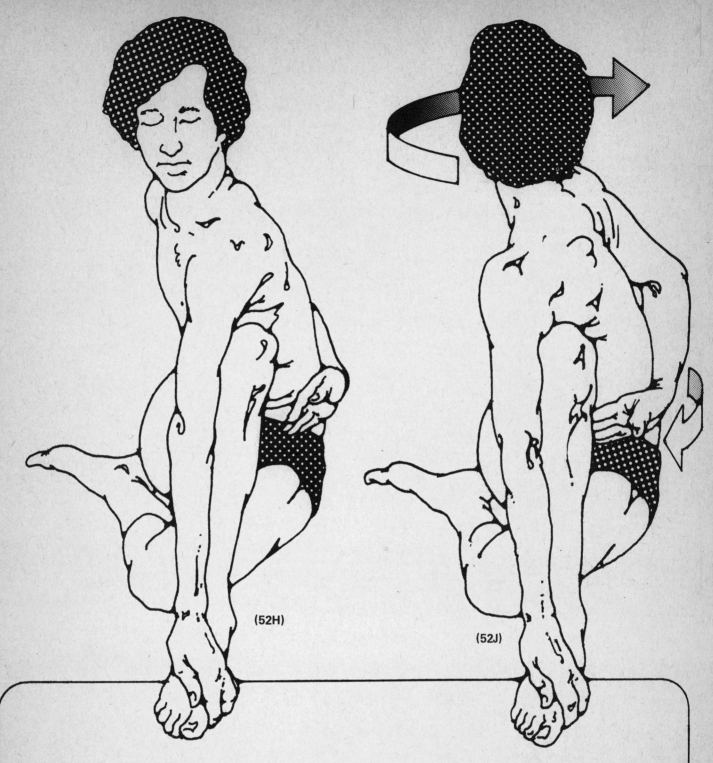

(52H)

(52J)

ARDHA MATSYENDRASAN/SPINE TWIST: *After you can do Position* **(52G)**, *without difficulty, lift the back hand up, wrapping it around your back so that it lies along your belly as in* **(52H, J)**. *Hold this position as previously stated, once on each side.*

This asan is highly beneficial and gives an unusual spiral twist to the entire spinal column. It also exercises the internal organs as well as limbering the hips and shoulders. People with slipped discs or back injuries should not do this asan unless they have checked with their doctor and are working under the close supervision of a qualified instructor. Do not jerk or snap the head around at any time during this exercise. Go in and out of the position slowly.

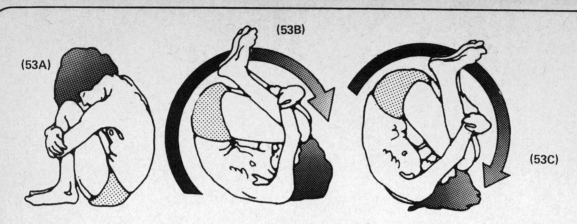

THE ROLL: *Clasp the arms around the knees and bring the forehead to the knees (53A). Now holding this position, roll backwards on the spine (ideally all the way up onto the shoulders and the back of the neck (53B, C). Then, maintaining your momentum, roll forward to the seated Position (53A). The Roll helps to make the spine flexible and limber and is a preparation for the Sarvangasan.*

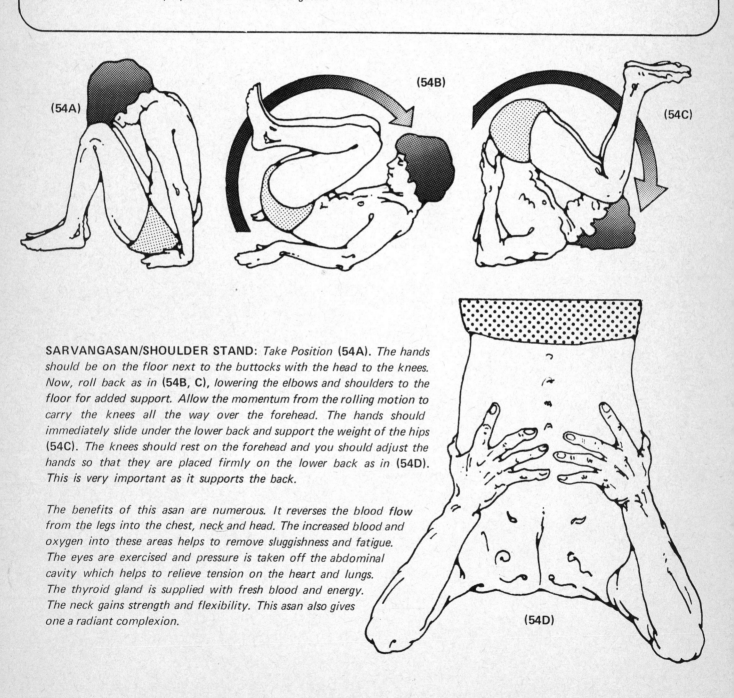

SARVANGASAN/SHOULDER STAND: *Take Position (54A). The hands should be on the floor next to the buttocks with the head to the knees. Now, roll back as in (54B, C), lowering the elbows and shoulders to the floor for added support. Allow the momentum from the rolling motion to carry the knees all the way over the forehead. The hands should immediately slide under the lower back and support the weight of the hips (54C). The knees should rest on the forehead and you should adjust the hands so that they are placed firmly on the lower back as in (54D). This is very important as it supports the back.*

The benefits of this asan are numerous. It reverses the blood flow from the legs into the chest, neck and head. The increased blood and oxygen into these areas helps to remove sluggishness and fatigue. The eyes are exercised and pressure is taken off the abdominal cavity which helps to relieve tension on the heart and lungs. The thyroid gland is supplied with fresh blood and energy. The neck gains strength and flexibility. This asan also gives one a radiant complexion.

48

The back of the neck should not be tense. Consciously relax the neck and shoulder muscles. Slowly begin to raise the legs away from the forehead **(54E)**, so that the knees are straight as in Position **(54F)**. You will notice that the support of your back becomes increasingly important. Then straighten the legs **(54G)**, so that your body forms a straight line from the shoulders to the feet. Again, relax the tension in your body. Once you have lifted into this position you should try to breathe gently and easily with the eyes wide open. Fix your gaze on the space between the big toes, which should be touching **(54G)**.

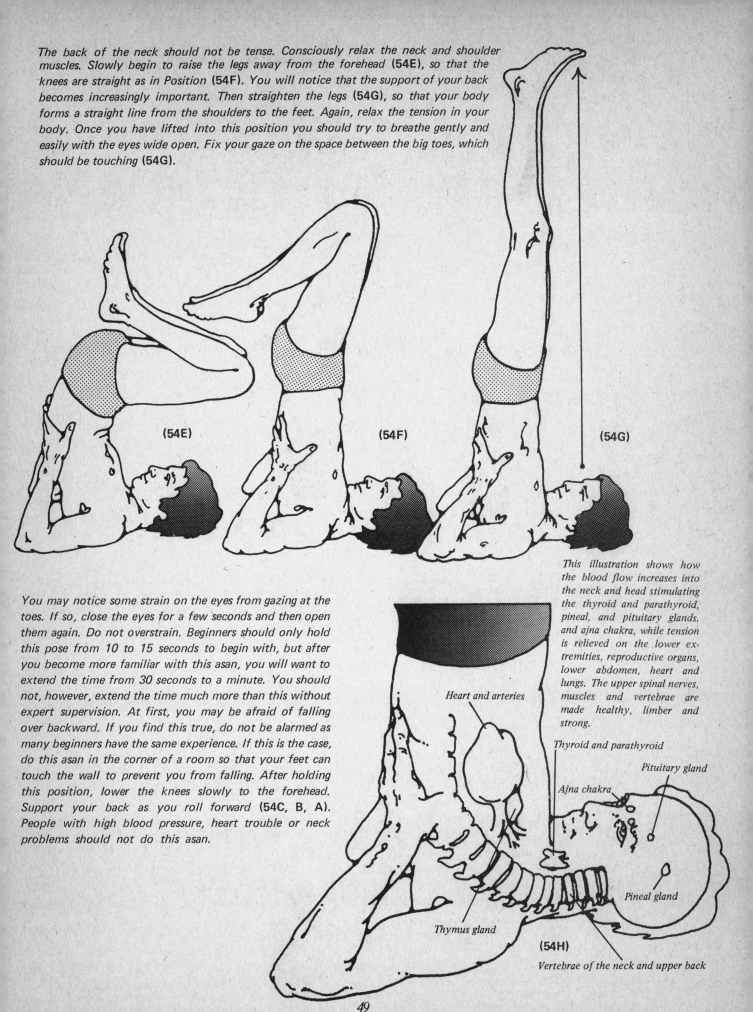

(54E)   **(54F)**   **(54G)**

You may notice some strain on the eyes from gazing at the toes. If so, close the eyes for a few seconds and then open them again. Do not overstrain. Beginners should only hold this pose from 10 to 15 seconds to begin with, but after you become more familiar with this asan, you will want to extend the time from 30 seconds to a minute. You should not, however, extend the time much more than this without expert supervision. At first, you may be afraid of falling over backward. If you find this true, do not be alarmed as many beginners have the same experience. If this is the case, do this asan in the corner of a room so that your feet can touch the wall to prevent you from falling. After holding this position, lower the knees slowly to the forehead. Support your back as you roll forward **(54C, B, A)**. People with high blood pressure, heart trouble or neck problems should not do this asan.

This illustration shows how the blood flow increases into the neck and head stimulating the thyroid and parathyroid, pineal, and pituitary glands, and ajna chakra, while tension is relieved on the lower extremities, reproductive organs, lower abdomen, heart and lungs. The upper spinal nerves, muscles and vertebrae are made healthy, limber and strong.

Heart and arteries

Thyroid and parathyroid

Pituitary gland

Ajna chakra

Pineal gland

Thymus gland

(54H)

Vertebrae of the neck and upper back

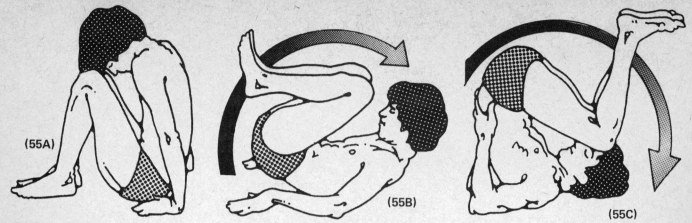

(55A)

(55B)

(55C)

HALASAN VARIATIONS/PLOW POSE: *You begin this asan in the same way as you do the Shoulder Stand. After you reach Position (55C), instead of lifting the legs up over the head, straighten them out and lower them down so that the toes are resting on the floor (55D). Keep the legs straight. Then, the hands can either remain supporting the back or lie palms down on the floor (55E). This puts a tremendous stretch on the back and legs. You will notice in (55D), that the toes are pointed toward the head and the heels are pressed gently to the floor. This puts a strong pull on the back of the legs and should be done gently. In Position (55E), the toes are pointed away from the head. This changes the pull slightly, stretching the back of the neck and spine. If you notice any headaches or unnecessary tension in the back of the neck and spine after doing this asan for a few days, you are putting undue strain on the nerves and muscles and should proceed more cautiously. This exercise along with the shoulder stand should not be done by people with nasal congestion or head colds as it will force the mucous into the brain and eye tissues. Women should not do this or the Shoulder Stand during the menstrual period.*

(55D)

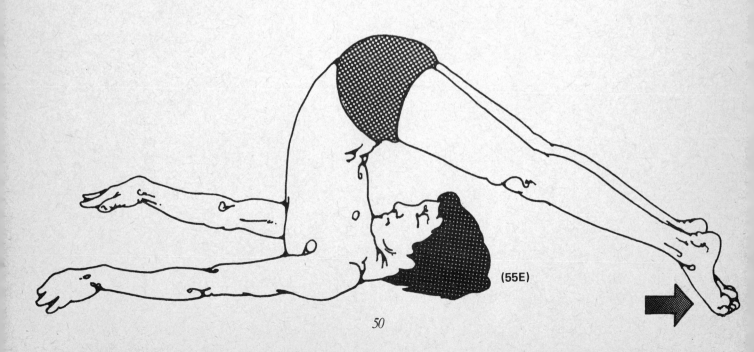

(55E)

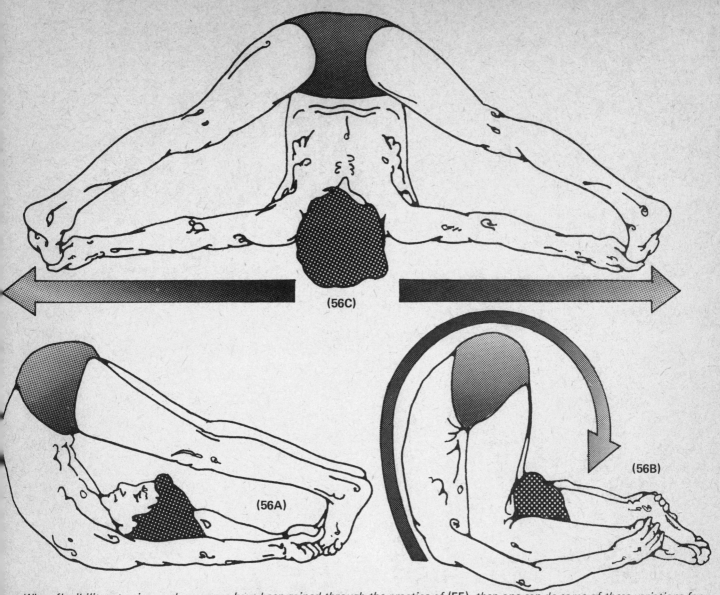

(56C)

(56A)

(56B)

When flexibility, stamina, and assurance have been gained through the practice of (55), then one can do some of these variations for increased benefits. (56A), bring the hands overhead from (55E) and grasp the toes. Press the heels toward the floor as far as possible. (56B), lower the knees down to the floor next to each ear. This is a difficult variation and demands maximum flexibility of the upper spine. (56C), hold onto the toes and spread the legs out as far as possible (56D), raise the arms straight off the floor from the shoulders. Keep the legs straight and raise the toes off the floor. You should be balancing on the shoulders and neck. This develops a beautiful complexion and clarity of mind.

When coming down out of these Plow Pose variations, you return the hands to the lower back for support and bring the knees to the forehead as in (55C). Then, supporting the back you roll forward (55B, A), and relax. At no time during the performance of this asan or the Shoulder Stand should you strain or try to go beyond your physical limitations. Use common sense and gentleness to gain maximum benefit from these asans.

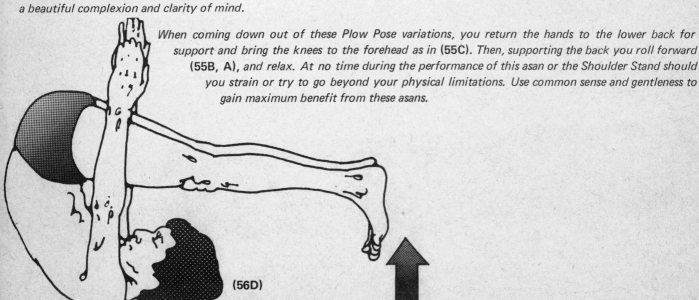

(56D)

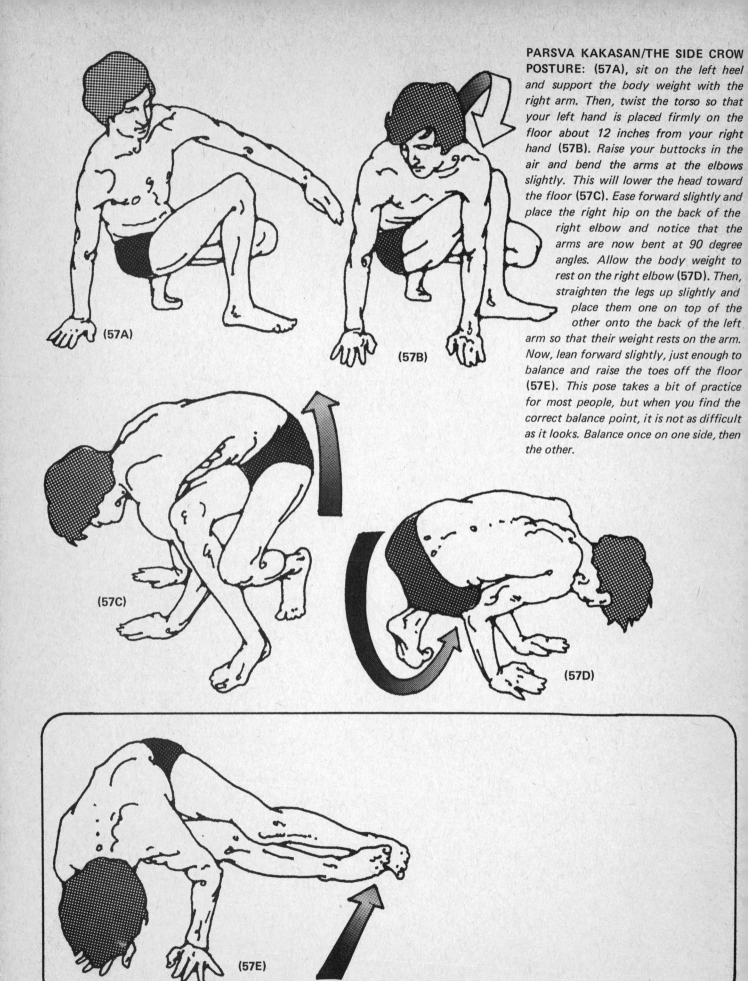

PARSVA KAKASAN/THE SIDE CROW POSTURE: (57A), *sit on the left heel and support the body weight with the right arm. Then, twist the torso so that your left hand is placed firmly on the floor about 12 inches from your right hand* **(57B).** *Raise your buttocks in the air and bend the arms at the elbows slightly. This will lower the head toward the floor* **(57C).** *Ease forward slightly and place the right hip on the back of the right elbow and notice that the arms are now bent at 90 degree angles. Allow the body weight to rest on the right elbow* **(57D).** *Then, straighten the legs up slightly and place them one on top of the other onto the back of the left arm so that their weight rests on the arm. Now, lean forward slightly, just enough to balance and raise the toes off the floor* **(57E).** *This pose takes a bit of practice for most people, but when you find the correct balance point, it is not as difficult as it looks. Balance once on one side, then the other.*

(57A)

(57B)

(57C)

(57D)

(57E)

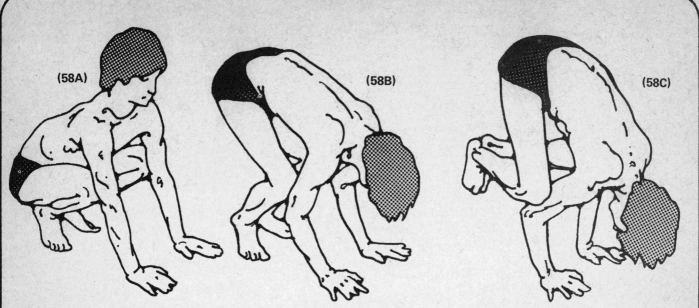

KAKASAN/CROW POSTURE: (58A), *crouch on your toes and hands. Spread the fingers apart like duck feet for better stability. Raise the buttocks in the air and lower the head toward the floor (58B). Then, place the knees firmly on the back of the elbows (notice that the arms are bent considerably in order to support the weight of the legs). Next, carefully lean forward, lowering the head toward the floor. Support the body weight on the hands, put the feet together and balance as long as possible (58C), breathing gently. Lower the toes and then the knees and relax. Caution: Keep your balance steady. Until you are sure of your steadiness use a pillow under your head to cushion you, should you slip.*

EASY SIRSHASAN/EASY HEADSTAND: *This is a headstand that is very simple and easy for most people. The full headstand should not be attempted unless one is working closely with a highly qualified instructor. You will want a folded blanket or something fairly soft under your head. Take Position (59A). With the top of your head on the floor, bend the elbows at right angles and place the hands firmly on the floor. Extend the legs straight in back, raising the buttocks in the air. Now, keeping the neck straight, raise the right knee and place it on the back of the right elbow. Place the left knee on the back of the left elbow. Then raise both feet off the floor and bring them together (59B). The spine and neck should be straight. Hold this position for a half minute or so if possible. If you experience dizziness or extreme pounding of the blood in the head come down immediately and take the baby pose (33B). If you have been noticing a strong pounding of the blood into the head in any of the inverted postures you should not try this headstand. Soon the arteries in the neck and head will become more elastic and this problem will be alleviated.*

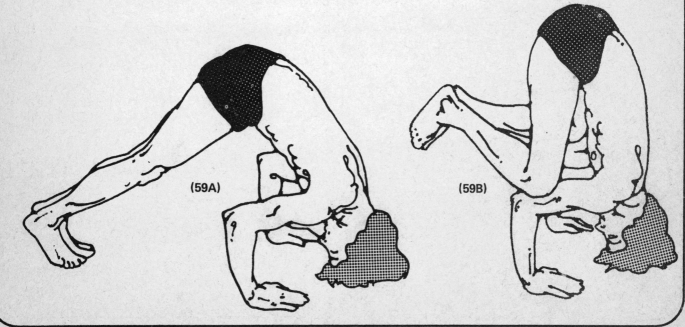

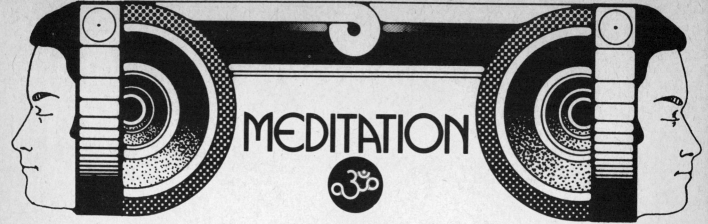

MEDITATION

In doing your asans and meditation poise the mind on the sound "OM," (pronounced "ohm"). Yogis believe that the universe is composed of various manifestations of sound. All of these manifestations are derived from the elemental sound OM (ॐ). It says in the Mandukya Upanishad: "OM—This imperishable sound is the whole of this universe. What has become, what is becoming and what will come—verily, all this is the sound OM. What is beyond these three states of the world of time—that too is verily OM." Repeat this sound to yourself mentally as you do the asans. Yogis find that by repeating OM mentally as they do their asans and meditation, that it not only increases the effectiveness of the asans, but makes the mind in meditation, vast, strong, pure, and still.

(60A)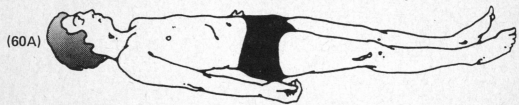

The art of relaxation and meditation is gaining widespread acceptance and practice by Americans these days. After every 2 or 3 asans depending upon their difficulty, one should take this pose (Savasan) for 30 to 90 seconds of complete relaxation. After you have finished your routine of Yoga postures, you should recline in this pose for 10 to 20 minutes of complete relaxation.

The science and experience of Yoga meditation (dhyana) is one that really must be learned with the aid of an experienced teacher; however, the relaxation technique is one that can be used to train beginners to still the mind and lead it safely and effectively in and out of Yoga meditation. In our more advanced manuals, we will go into this in detail, dealing with the various experiences, practices and their meanings. We feel that it is more important for beginners to have some practical experience rather than a multitude of various intellectual concepts that would mean nothing without the experience to back it up.

Not only is meditation a mental, emotional and spiritual experience, but it also has profound physiological effects. Many practitioners of Yoga meditation find that they become charged with electricity and energy through regular practice. Many find that physiological and mental problems cease to bother them and may disappear altogether. In reality the possibilities of dynamic, positive results from a regular practice of Yoga meditation (dhyana) yields benefits ranging from physiological improvements of nerves, glands, and health; increased mental clarity, perception and stability; to unbelievable powers of concentration, spiritual perfection and enlightenment of one's entire life and being.

Close your eyes and lie quietly in Savasan, so named because when one completely relaxes in this position the mind and senses are drawn inward into perfect stillness which leaves the body almost completely motionless. For a few minutes just lie there, breathing in and out deeply, without straining in any way. Let these ideas pass through the mind—"I don't have to speak for a few minutes. I don't have to move or respond to anyone or anything. For a few minutes I can become perfectly quiet in body and mind and I don't even have to think. I can become completely still and relaxed. I am not this body, nor am I this mind or intellect. I am something divine and free of all limitations. I am ageless, deathless, strong, ever free, eternally happy and pure." Now, begin to discharge all responsibilities. For a few minutes during your relaxation and meditation you should not be thinking of your family, bills, job, troubles, or even your name. The object is to unleash your mind from your duties, obligations, troubles, etc., allowing the mind to settle back into the immense stillness which surrounds and supports the mind and all of its functions and activities. In this way the body, mind, personality and what Yogis call the Atman, which is not the ego self, but rather the immortal, Divine Self, are charged, harmonized and cleansed.

To begin your relaxation bring your concentration or attention to the area of the forehead between the eyebrows and quietly imagine a diamondlike dot of light. This is a Yogic center of divine wisdom called the Ajna chakra. Now take your attention down your nose bone and across your eyebrows relaxing them. Let the force of gravity and your attention relax all of the muscles in the forehead and eyes and once they are relaxed don't allow them to flex until you want them to. Relax the whole face in this manner. Allow the eyes to sink back into the eye sockets until the muscles and nerves are completely stilled. This may take some practice, but it can and will be accomplished successfully. Now, picture your teeth, tongue and throat. "I don't have to speak at all for a few minutes." And now, relax the throat, tongue, teeth and the skin on the roof of the mouth. Take a deep breath, exhale and relax the lungs. As you do so, picture them in your mind's eye just as though they are bright and healthy, nourished and cleansed from your Yoga asans. Now, as you exhale, let them relax along with your entire ribcage and shoulder muscles. Picture the heart pumping nicely, steadily, day in and day out. Take a gentle deep breath and as you exhale let the heart relax. It doesn't have to beat so hard or fast now, just let it relax and carry on calmly. Picture your shoulders and arms, let them become empty and still. "I don't have to move my arms or hands for a few minutes." Picture the muscles and bones of the arm. Shake the arms and hands lightly and then let them fall, palms up next to the body. Let the hands become like gloves lying on a table with nothing inside, empty with no tension. Now, bring your attention to your belly. Picture all of your internal organs; stomach, intestines, kidneys, liver, etc. Let all of your insides settle back toward the floor free of all tension or strain. Now, simply observe the air moving in and out of the lungs through the nostrils. Do not try to hold the breath, stop it or speed it up, simply watch and observe what a wonderfully divine mechanism breathing is. "I don't have to breathe rapidly now, so my breathing can relax for a few minutes." Let your breathing become quiet, smooth, and free of all strain or tension. Picture the pelvis and let the bones, muscles, glands and nerves all become still and free of strain or tension. Picture the thigh muscles. Picture the bone running through the center of the thighs and then let the muscles and bones sink on the floor like warm putty or dough, no movement or tension. Continue all the way down the leg relaxing the knee joints, lower leg muscles, and ankles.

Picture the toes. Imagine that all of the tension and movement leave the toes and they become loose and still. Relax your heels where they touch the floor. Relax the floor. Now, bring your attention to the base of the spine at the tailbone. Picture how the spine is one blocklike bone on top of another, with a bright gold and silvery cord of electricity running up through the center of the bones right into the brain. Now, relax the spinal bones and nerves, releasing all tension, anxiety or fear all the way up from the base of the spine into the back of the neck. Picture where the brain and spinal cord touch at the back of the skull. Let this entire area become very loose and free of all tension, anxiety or stress. Move right into the brain itself and let it become absolutely quiet and unconcerned. Feel as though it relaxes and settles quietly in the skull. Gently bring your attention back to the space in the mind between the eyebrows. Without any anxiety, fear or strain, let the mind repeat the sound OM (see page 54). Let the mind simply play with the sound over and over for a few minutes. Then, let the mind become absolutely quiet and still, free of any movement, thought, remembrance, or imagination, perfectly still and quiet. Remain like this for ten minutes or so. As you come out of this state of relaxation and stillness, do not hurry or jerk. It is also very important that your mind is not jarred by harsh noises or interruptions while it is so quiet. For this reason you will want to find some quiet, undisturbed time for your relaxation and meditation. It is a good idea to take the phone off the hook before meditation. As you come out of your meditation, gently stretch as a cat does when it first wakes up. Breathe in gently and deeply. You will feel refreshed just as though you have had hours and hours of perfect rest. Then go about your day happily, healthfully and divinely.

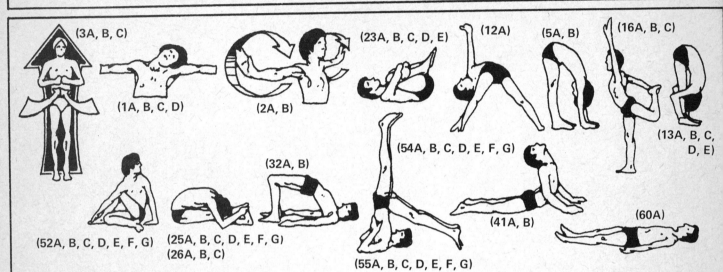

QUICK ROUTINE OF ESSENTIAL POSTURES: *After one has gained the initial benefits of a routine of Yoga exercises these postures should be done every day. I have set this routine up for those of you who might have a very busy and demanding schedule, but would still like a routine of exercises that could give you good benefits in 10 to 15 minutes.*

(16A, B, C)

(13A, B, C, D, E)

(54A, B, C, D, E, F, G)

(52A, B, C, E, F, G)

(55A, B, C, D, E, F, G)

(41A, B)

(60A)

(25A, B, C, D, E, F)

(3A, B, C)

(23A, B, C, D, E)

(12A)

(5A, B)

(16A, B, C)

(1A, B, C, D)

(2A, B)

(13A, B, C, D, E)

(54A, B, C, D, E, F, G)

(32A, B)

(41A, B)

(60A)

(52A, B, C, D, E, F, G)

(25A, B, C, D, E, F, G)
(26A, B, C)

(55A, B, C, D, E, F, G)

THE LIGHT ROUTINE: *This routine is for those of you who would like to have about 20 to 25 minutes of an easy work-out. This will provide the essential stretches, twists, and balances necessary for good health and clarity of mind, relieving stress for those individuals who have a very demanding schedule but would like to keep up their Yoga practice.*

There are approximately 75 asans and exercises in this manual. Under ordinary conditions and limitations we would expect one to be able to do all of the asans in this book correctly without strain within a year to a year-and-a-half. This will give those of you who are working on your own some idea of pacing and advancement. I have included a basic outline of a 6-week course that we use in our class setup. You might find it helpful to follow this for the first few months to get a safe, easy beginning to your Yoga practice.

FIRST WEEK
(1A, B, C, D); (2A, B); (3A, B, C,); (4A, B); (5A, B); (7A); (9A, B); (10A, B); (13A, B, C, D, E); (60A); (20A, B); (23A, B, C, D, E); (25A, B, C, D, E, F, G); (26A, B, C); (60A); (33A, B); (34A, B, C); (35A); and (60A).

SECOND WEEK
(1A, B, C, D); (2A, B); (3A, B, C); (6A, B, C); (8A, B, C); (9A, B); (10A, B,); (13A, B, C, D, E); (60 A); (20A, B); (22A, B); (23A, B, C, D, E); (25A, B, C, D, E, F, G); (26A, B, C); (60A); (30A, B); (32A, B); (33A, B); (34A, B, C); (35A); (41A, B); and (60A).

THIRD WEEK
This week do the same routine as the Second Week but add (40A, B), (45A, B) and (48A, B).

FOURTH WEEK
(1A, B, C, D); (2A, B); (3A, B, C); (5A, B); (10A, B); (11A); (13A, B, C, D, E); (15A, B); (60A); (16A, B, C); (25A, B, C, D, E, F, G); (26A, B, C); (32A, B); (39A, B); (40A, B); (45A, B); (52A, B, C, D, E, F, G); (41B); and (60A).

FIFTH WEEK
Continue routine of the Fourth Week, but add (53A, B, C), (54A, B, C, D, E, F, G); and (55A, B, C, D, E).

SIXTH WEEK
Continue Fourth and Fifth Week Routine adding (24A, B, C, D, E); (16D, E, F); (37A, B, C); and (38A, B).

(1A, B, C, D) HEAD ROTATIONS: *limbers and improves circulation in the muscles of the throat and the vertebrae of the neck.*

(2A, B) ARM ROTATIONS: *limbers shoulder joints, upper back muscles and nerves in the arms; improves circulation in the upper torso, neck and head.*

(3A, B, C) RAMA'S EASY POSE 1: *tones the central nervous system; helps to increase blood circulation.*

(4A, B) RAMA'S EASY POSE 2: *gives a light stretch to the muscles and nerves in the legs, back and neck; improves circulation of blood in the upper chest and head.*

(5A, B) PASCHIMOTTANASAN PREPARATION/FULL BEND *(literally means an intense stretch to the back of the entire body from head to heels): tones up and stretches the nervous system and muscle system from the heels to the back of the head, improves circulation of blood; strengthens the ribcage, lungs and heart muscles; helps to heal troubles of the sciatic nerves in the legs and varicose veins—great help for the diabetic.*

(6A, B, C) RAMA'S EASY POSE TWIST: *strengthens ankles and toes; improves blood circulation, expands chest and lungs; develops steadiness and poise.*

(7A) ALTERNATE LEG LIFT: *improves circulation of the urinary tract, the ovarian system and the gonads; strengthens legs; improves balance; removes fat from hips and thighs.*

(8A, B, C) COMPLETE LEG LIFT: *removes fatty deposits from thighs, hips, buttocks and waist; improves balance; strengthens the nerves and muscles in the legs.*

(9A, B) SVANASAN/STRETCHING DOG: *relieves exhaustion; limbers the tendons in the lower leg; limbers the shoulder joint relieving arthritis; relieves stress on the heart muscles and high*

blood pressure and rejuvenates the brain cells and eyes.

(10A, B) TRIKONA HASTHASAN/ALTERNATE TRIANGLE *(triangular stretch with the hands to the feet): localizes and stretches ligaments and nerves in the legs, back and neck; improves circulation in the entire pelvic region; removes fatty deposits in waist and exercises the intestines and kidneys; brings new blood to eyes and face.*

(11A, B, C) PRASARITA PADOTTANASAN/FULL TRIANGLE *(intense stretching of expanded legs): makes the hamstring and abductor muscles very strong; improves circulation and functioning of the kidneys, spleen, stomach, intestines, heart and lungs; rejuvenates brain cells.*

(12A) PARIVRITTA TRIKONASAN/TWISTING TRIANGLE *(twisting or revolving triangular posture: same as (11A, B, C); increases flexibility and blood circulation in the lower spine and pelvis, strengthens the hip joints; invigorates the abdominal viscera and diaphragm and strengthens the chest and neck; helps get rid of depression.*

(12B) UTTIHITA TRIKONASAN/SIDE TRIANGLE *(means intense, extended triangular stretch to the sides): tones the muscles of the legs and hips; stretches and develops the innercostal muscles of the ribcage; relieves backaches and strengthens the neck.*

(13A, B, C, D, E) PADAHASTHASAN/SUN POSE *(hands to feet, we also call this the Sun Pose for it is the first in the series of Surya Namaskar); all activities of the stomach, liver, spleen and abdominal regions are stimulated and improved; the tension and stress on the heart and lungs is relieved and the nerves and muscles of the entire back and legs are strengthened and limbered up; the blood is purified.*

(14A, B) PARSVOTTANASAN *(an intense stretching of the sides and chest): lubricates and limbers the shoulder joints and shoulder blades, lumbar vertebrae and neck; gives an intense stretch to the entire chest, lungs and heart; corrects breathing difficulties; tones the abdominal organs and strengthens the legs and back.*

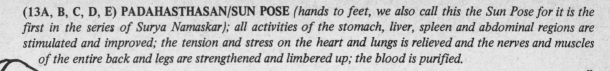

(15A, B) VRIKSASAN/TREE POSE: *strengthens legs, improves the concentration and balance; improves breathing.*

(15C, D, E, F, G) VRIKSASAN VARIATIONS: *same as (15A, B); strengthens knee joints.*

(16A, B, C) NATARAJASAN/THE DANCER POSE *(named after Lord Shiva, King of the Cosmic Dance of Creation, Preservation and Destruction): strengthens the lower back and lumbar vertebrae; stretches and strengthens the hips and thighs; improves balance, poise and concentration; removes phlegm and opens sinuses in the nasal passage; improves memory and gets rid of depression and sluggishness.*

(16E, F) VIRABHADRASAN *(named after the warrior son of Lord Shiva, Virabhadra): develops very strong legs and back; improves vigor and agility; tones the abdominal muscles and organs and increases concentration.*

(17A) VIRABHADRASAN VARIATION: *same as (16E, F); requires and develops excellent concentration, strengthens hips and pelvis.*

(17B) URDHVA PRASARITA EKAPADASAN/STORK STRETCH *(intense stretching, one leg with the opposite leg extended): removes fat from the waist, hips and legs, strengthens the nerves and muscles in legs considerably; good for diabetics.*

(18A, B, C, D) UTTIHITASAN *(extended stretch of the torso and hips: expands and stretches innercostal muscles of the ribcage; lines up the vertebrae in a correct position; relieves back strain.*

(19A) PADAHASTHANASAN VARIATION *(means hands to feet pose); localizes the stretch of the sciatic nerve; strengthens the hips and legs; increases blood circulation in the entire pelvic region.*

(20A, B) RAMA'S EASY POSE 3: *gives gentle, easy stretch to the sciatic nerves and muscles in the leg; tones the central nervous system; gives relief to varicose veins and bedsores; removes fat from thighs and hips.*

(21A, B) SUPTA PADANGUSTHASAN *(lying on the back grabbing the big toe): affords correct development and growth to the bones and muscles in the leg, relieving difficulties of sciatica and paralysis; rejuvenates nerves and muscles in the hips and pelvis.*

(22A, B) THE WALK: *removes fat from the abdomen, hips, buttocks and thighs; strengthens legs and eases constipation; strengthens the lower back.*

(23A, B, C, D, E) PAVANUMUKTASAN/KNEE SQUEEZE *(to relieve gas): relieves gas and bloaty sensation and heartburn in the entire abdominal region; increases blood circulation in head and neck; removes fat in abdomen and thighs.*

(24A, B, C, D) JATHARA PARIVARTANASAN *(a twisting motion of the abdomen and stomach):* tones up the activity and functioning of the liver, spleen, pancreas, stomach, kidneys, intestines; removes excess fat from the waist; strengthens the lower back and hips.

(25A, B, C, D, E, F, G and 26 A, B, C) PASCHIMOTTANASAN/SEATED SUN POSE *(literally means an intense stretch to the back of the entire body from head to heels):* helps to relieve constipation; strengthens the abdominal viscera and diaphram; increases digestive powers; and is excellent for diabetics; the sympathetic nervous system and the nerves in the leg are toned; the back and legs become very strong and supple; relieves impotency.

(27A, B, C, D) PASCHIMOTTANASAN VARIATION: *same benefits as (25) and (26); increases circulation of blood in the pelvis, gonads, ovaries, prostate, bladder and kidneys; strengthens the abdominal viscera; creates strong, supple legs; strengthens the back and hips.*

(28A, B) PADANGUSTHASAN/SPINE BALANCE *(means lifting to touch both toes):* strengthens abdominal viscera and all abdominal muscles and thigh muscles; improves balance and concentration; strengthens legs; relieves constipation and difficulties of the urinary tract.

(29A) MATSYASAN/FISH POSE *(named after the fish incarnation of Lord Vishnu, this variation is the Easy Fish):* the chest is fully expanded improving breathing and circulation; the lower back and neck become quite elastic; calcium deposits are removed from the spinal column; cures throat diseases; improves functioning of the thyroid glands; makes the eyes strong and bright.

(30A) ROWBOAT: *excellent for stretching and toning the muscles and nerves in the lower back and the inside of the thighs; increases flexibility of the spine; relieves sciatica and constipation; relieves impotency.*

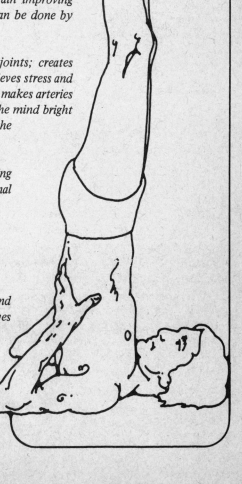

(31A, B, C) VIRASAN VARIATION/HERO POSTURE: *excellent for people with flat feet; cures stiffness in hips, knees and ankles; relieves bloatiness in the stomach and intestines; improves breathing and circulation in the entire pelvic region; tones the kidneys, uterine and ovarian systems and gonads; creates flexible lower back and hips; removes fat from the sides and thighs; relieves impotency.*

(32A, B) EASY BRIDGE: *improves the functioning of the thyroid and parathyroid glands thereby helping to improve functioning of the entire endocrine system; eases back pain and fatigue; increases blood circulation in the face and brain improving complexion and eyes; relieves hypertension; helps to cure bedsores; can be done by invalids in bed.*

(33A) VIRASAN/HERO POSE: *relieves stiffness in the knee joints; creates strong ankles and is beneficial for people with flat feet; (33B), relieves stress and fatigue; relieves headaches; relaxes the heart muscles and arteries; makes arteries and veins in the head, neck and chest elastic and strong; makes the mind bright and perceptive; gives clear bright eyes and good complexion — also called the Baby Pose due to the fetal position.*

(34A, B, C) and (36) SALABASAN VARIATIONS/LOCUST POSE *(resembling a locust):* strengthens the entire back and spinal column; increases abdominal pressure improving digestion and functioning of the vital organs.

(35A) POORVA NAVASAN/BOAT POSE: *same as (34A, B, C) and (36A).*

(37A, B, C) THE CAT BREATH: *increases the action of the intestines, heart, lungs, and liver; purifies the blood; relieves hypertension; limbers the spinal column and improves the entire breathing mechanism.*

(38A, B) LEG AND ARM BALANCE: *strengthens the hip joints; improves balance; promotes correct posture; strengthens the shoulders.*

(39A, B) DHANURASAN VARIATION/BOW POSTURE *(so named because this posture looks like a strung bow) strengthens the vertebrae, back muscles, hips. thighs, shoulders; improves balance and memory.*

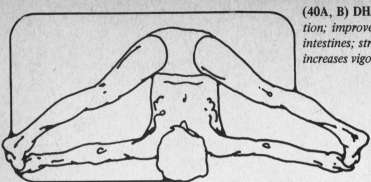

(40A, B) DHANURASAN/THE BOW POSTURE: *relieves chronic constipation; improves the functioning of the liver, kidneys, spleen, stomach and intestines; strengthens the back and thighs; aligns the vertebrae properly and increases vigor and vitality.*

(41A, B) BHUJANGASAN/COBRA POSE *(resembles the movement of a cobra): improves the working of the intestines; increases body heat; helps to awaken kundalini; forces equal amount of energy and electricity into each side of the brain; tones the ovaries and uterus, and gonads; increases overall body strength; relieves impotency.*

(42A, B) UTTIHITA VIRASAN/HERO POSE EXTENSION: *increases blood to the head; purifies and oxygenates the blood; strengthens the shoulders, chest, ankles and knees.*

(43A, B, C) SVANASAN/THE STRETCHING DOG POSE: *the innercostal muscles of the ribcage are strengthened; the muscles of the chest, neck, abdomen, and groin are made elastic and strong; the pelvic region receives an increased amount of blood which improves all functioning of nerves and organs in that region, relieving impotency; strengthens back and leg muscles and nerves; reduces body fat.*

(44A, B, C,) HANUMANASAN PREPARATION *(named after Hanuman, the great devotee of Lord Rama); strengthens the abductor muscles of the thighs and hips; increases the pelvic blood circulation; tones the pelvic nerves; relieves impotency; elongates the nerves and muscles of the legs.*

(45A, B) HIPS AND KNEES: *makes the knees, hips, ankles and lower back strong, supple, and capable of doing more difficult asans.*

(46A, B, C, D) PADMASAN PREPARATION/LOTUS POSE PREPARATION: *elongates the spinal nerves and spinal cord and the muscles of the spinal column; strengthens the hips, knees and ankles; elongates the thigh muscles and sciatic nerve; makes possible the full Padmasan and other more difficult asans.*

(47A, B) MOUNTAIN POSE PREPARATION: *same as (46A, B, C, D); strengthens thighs and knees.*

(48A, B) BHADRASAN/THRONE OF SHIVA *(so named for it is an advanced seated pose used by ascetics and worshippers of Lord Shiva): helps check irregular menstrual activity; excellent for women in the first 3 to 5 months of pregnancy to strengthen the hip joints and pelvic nerves and muscles for easier delivery; relieves urinary difficulties; prevents susceptibility to hernia; and tones the prostate gland; tones the reproductive nerves relieving impotency.*

(49A, B) SHIVA SHAKTIASAN/DIAMOND POSE *(named after Lord Shiva and his Shakti, or Power, because it forms 2 intersecting triangles): tones the entire electrical system from the base of the spine to the top of the head; strengthens and elongates the sciatic nerves; improves digestion and strengthens the hip joints.*

(50A, B, C, D) and (51A) RAJAKAPOTASAN/PIGEON POSTURE: *rejuvenates the sacral lumbar and cervical vertebrae of the spine; affords maximum strength of the hip joints; makes the back and neck very strong; activates the adrenals and gonads, thyroid and parathyroid glands; increases vitality; relieves impotency; and strengthens the ribcage and chest; improves functioning of the reproductive nerves and organs.*

(52A, B, C, D, E, F, G, H, J) ARDHA MATSYENDRASAN/SPINE TWIST *(named after the Lord of the Fishes, Matsyendra, who was a great devotee of Lord Shiva and who was responsible for much of Hatha Yoga Science as we know it today): cures chronic constipation, and urinary and bladder difficulties; helps awaken kundalini; affords maximum lateral movement of the vertebrae; relieves prostate difficulties; improves digestion; tones the nerves of the spine from the base of the pelvis up into the brain and eyes.*

(54A, B, C, D, E, F, G, H) SARVANGASAN/SHOULDER STAND *(the whole body pose): one of the greatest of all asans for modern man; tones the entire endocrine system through its beneficial and dynamic effects on the thyroid and parathyroid glands in the neck; relieves impotency and enhances the functioning of all vital organs; helps to relieve many respiratory difficulties; soothes the entire nervous system; relieves constipation and epilepsy; removes fatigue; makes the mind bright and clear; relieves hypertension; improves eyesight and helps to activate the ajna chakra, the yogic center of divine wisdom between the eyebrows.*

(55A, B, C, D, E) HALASAN/PLOW POSE: *tones up the thyroid and parathyroid gland, improving glandular functioning of the entire body; gives a complete stretch to the spinal cord, nerves and muscles and the muscles and nerves of the legs; relieves hypertension; constipation; muscular rheumatism and lumbago; reduces body fat, and enlargement of the liver and spleen are relieved; affords excellent blood supply to the nerve ganglion of the spinal cord and prevents ossification of the vertebrae and dowager's hump; relieves high blood pressure; makes the arteries and veins supple, elastic and strong.* **(56A, B)** *affords maximum bend and elasticity to the legs and exercises the internal organs;* **(56D),** *creates radiant complexion and eyes, cures drooping shoulders.*

(57A, B, C, D, E) PARSWA KAKASAN/SIDE CROW POSTURE: *strengthens the arms, shoulders, wrists, hands; improves functioning of the intestines; stomach, heart and lungs; tones the sinus cavities in the nasal passage; makes the spine elastic and strong and improves balance.*

(58A, B, C) KAKASAN: *strengthens hands, wrists, arms and shoulders; improves balance and relieves tension on the heart and arteries.*

(59A, B) EASY SIRSHASAN/EASY HEADSTAND: *improves and insures complete blood circulation in the head, neck and chest; strengthens neck and shoulders, relieves hypertension and constipation; improves mental clarity; affords a sense of well-being; can be done safely without the dangers of the full headstand.*

(60A) SAVASAN/CORPSE POSE: *this asan removes any fatigue or strain produced by the other asans, work, or stress of the day.*

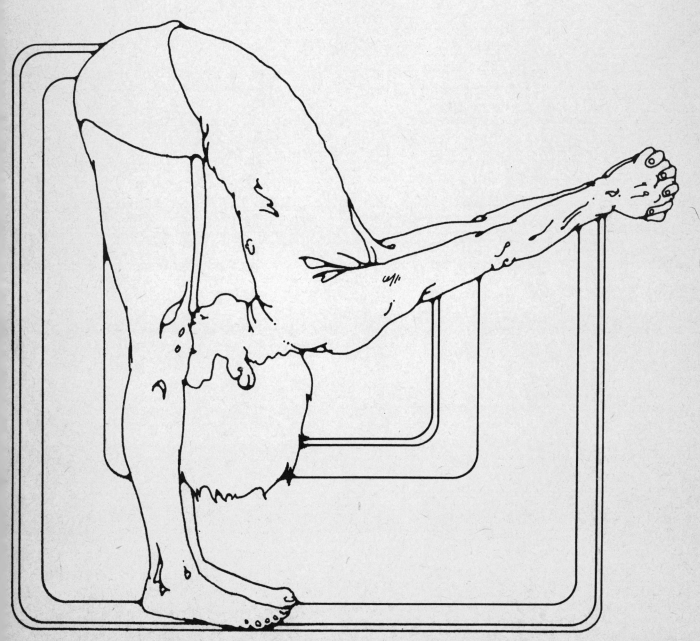